FATTY LIVER
DIET COOKBOOK
FOR
NEWLY DIAGNOSED

A Comprehensive Guide with Nutritious
Recipes to Revitalize Your Liver
Including Easy-to-Follow 30-Day Meal
Plan to Achieve Optimal Well-being

KELLY C. BROWN

CONTENTS

INTRODUCTION

Clara received devastating news about her being diagnosed with fatty liver disease. She was overtaken with shock and panic, but she knew she had to fight back. That's when she came across a cookbook that would save her life.

Clara felt herself attracted into a world of vivid, tasty, and healthy meals as she leafed through the pages of the guidebook. Each page held out the prospect of a brighter, healthier future. It was a healing journey via the art of cooking.

Clara set off on her culinary adventure with determination in her heart. She turned her kitchen into a wellness laboratory, stocked with fresh products and recipes that claimed to heal her liver. Her debut recipe was a vibrant kale salad with a tangy lemon vinaigrette. It was a revelation; each bite was a jolt of energy.

Clara's kitchen trials continued as the weeks evolved into months. She perfected the knack of cooking luscious fish, relishing the omega-3 fatty acids that supported her rehabilitation.

Her friends and family admired her increased abilities, unaware that each meal was a modest victory over her condition.

Clara's vigor returned as her rehabilitation progressed. She gained energy, and her liver function tests revealed positive results. Friends and coworkers couldn't help but inquire about her secret. Clara handed each of them a copy of the cookbook that had been her lifeline, a glimmer of hope in her eyes.

Clara's path from a life-altering illness to a life full of health and vigor began simply, but profoundly, within the pages of a cookbook. It was a narrative of grit, empowerment, and the transformational power of food.

Clara's narrative, in the end, was more than simply about her own recovery; it was a beacon of hope for countless others facing a similar battle. She inspired others to take care of their health, one tasty and healthy meal at a time, through the cookbook that had saved her life.

Welcome on the path to a healthier liver! Adopting a balanced and healthy diet is critical to controlling and possibly correcting fatty liver disease if you've recently been diagnosed. This Fatty Liver Diet Cookbook is your guide to delectable, liver-friendly foods designed to improve your health. These dishes, which are packed with nutrient-rich foods and conscious culinary decisions, seek to minimize fat deposition in the liver while providing a fulfilling and flavorful culinary experience.

Allow this cookbook to be your partner on the journey to greater liver health, with a diverse assortment of foods that prioritize flavor without jeopardizing your commitment to liver care. Accept this culinary adventure and allow the healing power of wholesome, carefully selected ingredients to improve your approach to food and wellness.

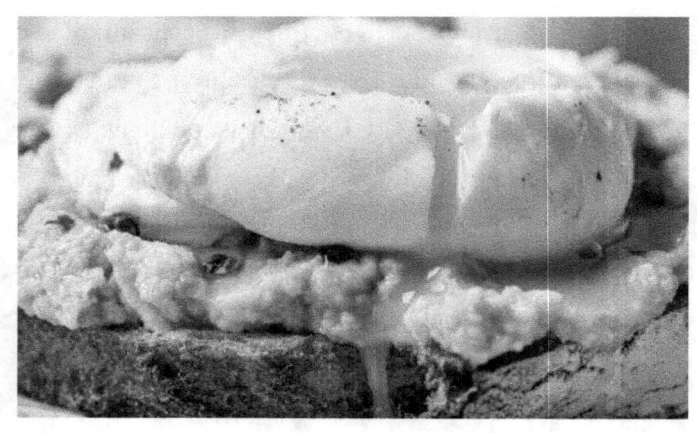

"My body is healing, and I
am committed to my
well-being."

CHAPTER 1: WHAT IS FATTY LIVER?

Fatty liver disease, also known as hepatic steatosis, is a disorder in which excess fat accumulates in the liver cells. If left untreated, this fat deposition can compromise normal liver function and lead to more serious liver issues.

TYPES OF FATTY LIVER DISEASE

1. NAFLD (Non-Alcoholic Fatty Liver Disease):

Causes: NAFLD is caused mostly by other reasons than alcohol consumption. The precise reason is not always obvious, however it is frequently associated with:

- Obesity: Excess body fat, particularly around the belly, is a major risk factor.
- Insulin Resistance: When the cells in the body do not respond adequately to insulin, fat accumulates in the liver.
- Metabolic Syndrome (MS): A group of disorders that includes excessive blood pressure, diabetes, and abnormal cholesterol levels.
- Type 2 Diabetes: Diabetics are at a higher risk.

- Genetics: Certain hereditary factors can predispose people to NAFLD.

NAFLD can proceed through several stages:

- Simple Steatosis: Is defined as fat buildup in the liver without considerable inflammation or damage to the liver cells.
- Non-Alcoholic Steatohepatitis (NASH): It's characterized by fat accumulation, inflammation, and liver cell damage. NASH is more serious since it can progress to fibrosis and cirrhosis.
- Fibrosis and Cirrhosis: As NASH advances, it can cause liver scarring (fibrosis) and, eventually, cirrhosis, which is extensive liver scarring that inhibits liver function.

2. AFLD (Alcoholic Fatty Liver Disease):

Causes: Excessive and persistent alcohol use causes AFLD. Even modest alcohol use can lead to this illness over time.

AFLD includes stages as well:

- Alcoholic Fatty Liver: The first stage is distinguished by fat accumulation in liver cells.

- Alcoholic Hepatitis: Liver inflammation caused by alcohol damage. The symptoms might be rather severe.
- Cirrhosis: Chronic alcohol usage can develop in cirrhosis, which is extensive liver scarring that can lead to liver failure.

SYMPTOMS

1. Fatty liver disease is frequently asymptomatic, particularly in the early stages.
2. In severe stages, symptoms may include weariness, stomach discomfort, and yellowing of the skin and eyes (jaundice).

WHY DIET MATTERS

Diet is critical in the management of fatty liver disease, especially for those who have recently been diagnosed.

Here's why it's important:

1. Weight Management: Obesity is frequently connected with fatty liver disease. A good diet can help you control your weight, which can prevent fat deposition in the liver.

2. Reduced Fat Intake: It is critical to restrict your intake of saturated and trans fats, which can aggravate liver inflammation. A well-balanced diet can assist you in reducing these harmful fats.

3. Sugar Consumption Management: Fatty liver disease can be exacerbated by a high sugar diet, particularly from added sugars and sugary beverages. A low-sugar diet can help manage the illness.

4. Increased Fiber: Consuming foods high in fiber, such as fruits, vegetables, and whole grains, can help manage blood sugar levels and minimize fat deposition in the liver.

5. Balanced Macronutrients: To promote general health and liver function, consume a variety of carbs, proteins, and healthy fats.

6. Restrict Alcohol: If you drink alcohol, you should restrict or eliminate it because it might worsen liver damage in people with fatty liver disease.

7. Nutrient-Rich Foods: Focus on nutrient-dense foods such as lean meats, leafy greens, and antioxidant-rich meals to enhance liver function.

8. Portion Control: Control your portion sizes to avoid overeating, which can contribute to weight gain and aggravate fatty liver.

9. Hydration: Keeping hydrated is critical for liver function. Throughout the day, drink lots of water.

FOODS TO EAT AND FOODS TO AVOID

FOODS TO EAT

1. Fruits and Vegetables: Consume a variety of colored fruits and vegetables, such as berries, apples, spinach, kale, and broccoli. They are high in fiber and antioxidants.

2. Whole Grains: Choose whole grains such as brown rice, quinoa, and whole wheat bread. They include more fiber and minerals than processed grains.

3. Lean Proteins: Choose lean protein sources such as skinless poultry, fish, tofu, and legumes (beans, lentils, chickpeas).

4. Healthy Fats: Avocados, almonds, seeds, and olive oil are all good sources of healthful fats. These lipids are beneficial to the liver.

5. Low-Fat Dairy: Choose low-fat or fat-free dairy products such as yogurt and milk.

6. Herbal Teas: Herbal teas, such as green tea and dandelion tea, may be healthy to the liver.

7. Water: Drink plenty of water throughout the day to stay hydrated.

FOODS TO AVOID

1. Sugary Foods: Sugary meals and beverages, such as sodas, sweets, and sugary cereals, should be avoided.

2. Processed Foods: Processed meals, such as fast food, chips, and pre-packaged snacks, are rich in trans fats and should be avoided.

3. High-Fructose Corn Syrup: Check labels for high-fructose corn syrup, which is found in many processed foods and sugary drinks.

4. Saturated and Trans Fats: Limit your consumption of foods high in saturated fats, such as fatty cuts of meat and full-fat dairy. Avoid trans fats, which are commonly present in fried foods and some margarines.

5. Excessive Salt: Limit your intake of high-sodium foods, as they might contribute to fluid retention and inflammation.

6. Alcohol: Limit or avoid alcohol usage because it can aggravate liver damage.

7. Red Meat: Reduce your intake of red meat, particularly processed and fatty slices.

8. Refined Grains and White Bread: Choose whole grains over refined grains such as white bread and white rice.

SHOPPING LIST FOR FATTY LIVER DIET

A Fatty Liver Diet shopping list includes nutrient-dense items that enhance liver function while limiting saturated fats and added sugars.

Here's a comprehensive shopping list to help you:

1. **Lean Proteins:**
   ○ Skinless poultry (chicken or turkey)
   ○ Fish (salmon, mackerel, trout)
   ○ Lean cuts of meat (such as sirloin or tenderloin)

2. **Plant-Based Proteins:**
   - Legumes (lentils, chickpeas, black beans)
   - Tofu and tempeh
   - Quinoa
3. **Fruits:**
   - Berries (blueberries, strawberries, raspberries)
   - Citrus fruits (oranges, grapefruits, lemons)
   - Apples and pears
4. **Vegetables:**
   - Leafy greens (spinach, kale, collard greens)
   - Cruciferous vegetables (broccoli, cauliflower, Brussels sprouts)
   - Colorful vegetables (bell peppers, carrots, tomatoes)
5. **Whole Grains:**
   - Brown rice
   - Whole wheat bread or pasta
   - Oats and barley
6. **Healthy Fats:**
   - Avocado

- Nuts (almonds, walnuts)
- Olive oil

7. **Dairy or Dairy Alternatives:**
   - Low-fat or fat-free yogurt
   - Almond or soy milk

8. **Herbs and Spices:**
   - Turmeric
   - Garlic
   - Ginger
   - Cinnamon

9. **Beverages:**
   - Green tea
   - Water (stay hydrated)

10. **Avoid or Limit:**
    - Processed foods
    - Sugary beverages
    - Fried and fast foods
    - Excessive red meat

11. **Snacks:**
    - Hummus with veggie sticks
    - Fresh fruit
    - Air-popped popcorn

"I make nourishing choices that support my liver's health."

"Every healthy meal I eat brings me closer to optimal liver function."

CHAPTER 2: 30-DAY MEAL PLAN

Dive into each chapter recipes to learn about the ingredients and step-by-step directions for preparation, allowing you to easily embark on a month-long journey of nutrients and flavor to revive your liver health.

DAY 1

Breakfast: Oatmeal with berries and almonds

Lunch: Grilled chicken salad with mixed greens and olive oil dressing

Snack: Greek yogurt with sliced cucumber

Dinner: Baked salmon with quinoa and steamed broccoli

DAY 2

Breakfast: Whole grain toast with avocado and poached eggs

Lunch: Lentil soup with a side of mixed vegetables

Snack: Handful of cherry tomatoes with mozzarella cheese

Dinner: Turkey meatballs with whole grain pasta and roasted asparagus

DAY 3

Breakfast: Smoothie with spinach, banana, and chia seeds

Lunch: Quinoa salad with cherry tomatoes, feta cheese, and olive oil

Snack: Apple slices with almond butter

Dinner: Grilled cod with quinoa and roasted Brussels sprouts

DAY 4

Breakfast: Greek yogurt parfait with granola and mixed berries

Lunch: Stir-fried tofu with broccoli and brown rice

Snack: Carrot and celery sticks with hummus

Dinner: Grilled shrimp with quinoa and sautéed spinach

DAY 5

Breakfast: Whole grain pancakes with sliced strawberries

Lunch: Chickpea salad with cherry tomatoes, cucumber, and lemon-tahini dressing

Snack: Cottage cheese with pineapple chunks

Dinner: Baked chicken breast with quinoa pilaf and steamed broccoli

DAY 6

Breakfast: Scrambled eggs with spinach and whole grain toast

Lunch: Turkey and vegetable wrap with whole wheat tortilla

Snack: Mixed nuts and dried fruits

Dinner: Baked tilapia with wild rice and steamed asparagus

DAY 7

Breakfast: Overnight oats with almond milk, chia seeds, and sliced peaches

Lunch: Quinoa-stuffed bell peppers with black beans and corn

Snack: Sliced mango with a squeeze of lime

Dinner: Stir-fried tofu with broccoli, bell peppers, and brown rice

DAY 8

Breakfast: Avocado and tomato omelet with whole grain toast

Lunch: Spinach and feta stuffed chicken breast with quinoa

Snack: Edamame beans with a sprinkle of sea salt

Dinner: Grilled vegetable and tofu skewers with couscous

DAY 9

Breakfast: Berry and kale smoothie with a scoop of protein powder

Lunch: Lentil and vegetable curry with brown rice

Snack: Sliced bell peppers with guacamole

Dinner: Baked cod with lemon-dill sauce, sweet potato, and green beans

DAY 10

Breakfast: Whole grain waffles with Greek yogurt and sliced banana

Lunch: Turkey and vegetable stir-fry with brown rice

Snack: Handful of cherry tomatoes with mozzarella cheese

Dinner: Quinoa-stuffed acorn squash with roasted Brussels sprouts

DAY 11

Breakfast: Chia seed pudding with mixed berries

Lunch: Caprese salad with whole grain crackers

Snack: Greek yogurt with sliced cucumber

Dinner: Grilled salmon with quinoa pilaf and steamed broccoli

DAY 12

Breakfast: Whole grain English muffin with scrambled eggs and sliced avocado

Lunch: Chickpea and vegetable wrap with a side of mixed greens

Snack: Cottage cheese with pineapple chunks

Dinner: Baked chicken thighs with sweet potato mash and green beans

DAY 13

Breakfast: Banana and almond butter smoothie with a handful of spinach

Lunch: Shrimp and vegetable kebabs with whole grain couscous

Snack: Mixed nuts and dried cranberries

Dinner: Turkey chili with black beans, tomatoes, and a side of whole grain rice

DAY 14

Breakfast: Overnight oats with almond milk, chia seeds, and sliced peaches

Lunch: Mediterranean-style grilled chicken salad with olives and feta

Snack: Sliced cucumber with tzatziki sauce

Dinner: Baked cod with lemon-dill sauce, sweet potato, and green beans

DAY 15

Breakfast: Whole grain bagel with smoked salmon, cream cheese, and capers

Lunch: Quinoa and black bean bowl with avocado and salsa

Snack: Sliced mango with a squeeze of lime

Dinner: Stir-fried tofu with broccoli, bell peppers, and brown rice

DAY 16

Breakfast: Greek yogurt parfait with granola and mixed berries

Lunch: Spinach and mushroom omelet with a side of whole grain toast

Snack: Apple slices with almond butter

Dinner: Baked chicken breast with quinoa pilaf and steamed broccoli

DAY 17
Breakfast: Whole grain pancakes with sliced strawberries
Lunch: Lentil and vegetable soup with a whole grain roll
Snack: Carrot and celery sticks with hummus
Dinner: Grilled shrimp with quinoa and sautéed spinach

DAY 18
Breakfast: Scrambled eggs with spinach and whole grain toast
Lunch: Turkey and vegetable stir-fry with brown rice
Snack: Mixed nuts and dried fruits
Dinner: Baked salmon with quinoa and steamed broccoli

DAY 19
Breakfast: Smoothie with spinach, banana, and chia seeds
Lunch: Quinoa salad with cherry tomatoes, feta cheese, and olive oil
Snack: Greek yogurt with sliced cucumber

Dinner: Grilled cod with quinoa and roasted Brussels sprouts

DAY 20

Breakfast: Avocado and tomato omelet with whole grain toast

Lunch: Chickpea and vegetable curry with quinoa

Snack: Sliced bell peppers with guacamole

Dinner: Grilled chicken with wild rice and steamed asparagus

DAY 21

Breakfast: Greek yogurt with sliced banana and a handful of walnuts

Lunch: Turkey and vegetable wrap with whole wheat tortilla

Snack: Cottage cheese with pineapple chunks

Dinner: Baked tilapia with wild rice and steamed asparagus

DAY 22

Breakfast: Berry and kale smoothie with a scoop of protein powder

Lunch: Lentil and vegetable curry with brown rice

Snack: Handful of cherry tomatoes with mozzarella cheese

Dinner: Beef and vegetable kebabs with sweet potato wedges

DAY 23

Breakfast: Whole grain waffles with Greek yogurt and sliced banana

Lunch: Quinoa-stuffed bell peppers with black beans and corn

Snack: Mixed nuts and dried cranberries

Dinner: Baked cod with lemon-dill sauce, sweet potato, and green beans

DAY 24

Breakfast: Chia seed pudding with mixed berries

Lunch: Spinach and feta stuffed chicken breast with quinoa

Snack: Edamame beans with a sprinkle of sea salt

Dinner: Grilled vegetable and tofu skewers with couscous

DAY 25

Breakfast: Banana and almond butter smoothie with a handful of spinach

Lunch: Shrimp and vegetable kebabs with whole grain couscous

Snack: Mixed nuts and dried apricots

Dinner: Turkey chili with black beans, tomatoes, and a side of whole grain rice

DAY 26

Breakfast: Avocado and egg breakfast burrito with salsa on a whole wheat tortilla

Lunch: Quinoa and black bean bowl with avocado and salsa

Snack: Sliced cucumber with tzatziki sauce

Dinner: Baked chicken thighs with sweet potato mash and green beans

DAY 27

Breakfast: Whole grain English muffin with scrambled eggs and sliced avocado

Lunch: Mediterranean-style grilled chicken salad with olives and feta

Snack: Sliced mango with a squeeze of lime

Dinner: Stir-fried tofu with broccoli, bell peppers, and brown rice

DAY 28

Breakfast: Greek yogurt parfait with granola and mixed berries

Lunch: Spinach and mushroom omelet with a side of whole grain toast

Snack: Apple slices with almond butter

Dinner: Baked chicken breast with quinoa pilaf and steamed broccoli

DAY 29

Breakfast: Whole grain pancakes with sliced strawberries

Lunch: Lentil and vegetable soup with a whole grain roll

Snack: Carrot and celery sticks with hummus

Dinner: Grilled shrimp with quinoa and sautéed spinach

DAY 30

Breakfast: Scrambled eggs with spinach and whole grain toast

Lunch: Turkey and vegetable stir-fry with brown rice

Snack: Mixed nuts and dried fruits

Dinner: Baked salmon with quinoa and steamed broccoli

"I am in control of my health, and I choose wellness."

"I am grateful for the opportunity to heal and improve my liver health."

CHAPTER 3: BREAKFAST RECIPES

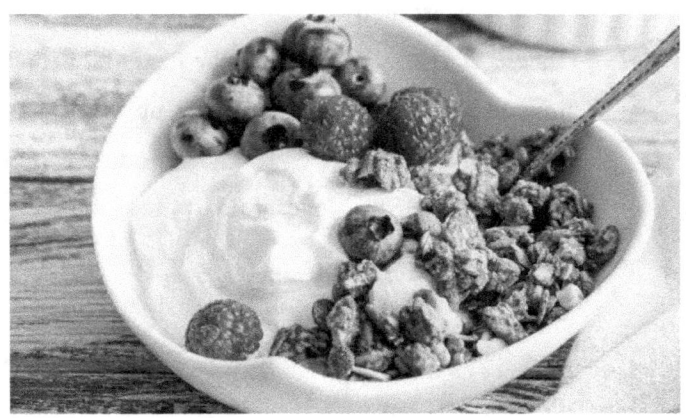

Oatmeal with berries and almonds

Ingredients:

- 1/2 cup rolled oats
- 1 cup milk (dairy or plant-based)
- A handful of mixed berries (such as strawberries, blueberries, raspberries)
- 2 tablespoons sliced almonds
- 1 tablespoon honey or maple syrup (optional, for sweetness)
- A pinch of cinnamon (optional, for flavor)

Instructions:

1. In a saucepan, combine the rolled oats and milk. Bring it to a gentle boil over medium heat, stirring occasionally.

2. Once it starts boiling, reduce the heat to low and simmer for about 5-7 minutes or until the oats are cooked and have reached your desired consistency. Stir occasionally to prevent sticking.

3. While the oatmeal is cooking, wash and prepare the berries. If using larger berries like strawberries, you may want to slice them.

4. Once the oatmeal is ready, remove it from the heat and transfer it to a serving bowl.

5. Top the oatmeal with the mixed berries and sliced almonds.

6. Drizzle honey or maple syrup over the top for added sweetness, if desired.

7. Sprinkle a pinch of cinnamon over the oatmeal for extra flavor.

8. Give it a gentle stir to combine the ingredients.

Whole grain toast with avocado and poached eggs

Ingredients:

- 2 slices of whole grain bread
- 1 ripe avocado
- 2 large eggs
- Salt and pepper to taste
- Optional toppings: red pepper flakes, chives, or a squeeze of lemon juice

Instructions:

1. Toast the whole grain bread slices to your liking.
2. While the bread is toasting, cut the avocado in half, remove the pit, and scoop the flesh into a bowl. Mash the avocado with a fork and season with salt and pepper.
3. Poach the eggs by bringing a pot of water to a gentle simmer. Crack each egg into a separate small bowl and carefully slide them into the simmering water. Cook for about 3-4 minutes for a runny yolk.
4. While the eggs are poaching, spread the mashed avocado evenly on the toasted bread slices.

5. Once the eggs are poached, carefully remove them from the water with a slotted spoon and place one on each slice of avocado-covered toast.

6. Sprinkle with additional salt and pepper to taste, and add any optional toppings like red pepper flakes, chives, or a squeeze of lemon juice.

Smoothie with spinach, banana, and chia seeds

Ingredients:

- 1 cup fresh spinach leaves, washed
- 1 ripe banana
- 1 tablespoon chia seeds
- 1/2 cup Greek yogurt
- 1/2 cup almond milk (or any preferred milk)
- 1 teaspoon honey (optional, for sweetness)
- Ice cubes (optional)

Instructions:

1. Place the fresh spinach leaves in a blender.
2. Peel the ripe banana and add it to the blender.
3. Spoon in the chia seeds, Greek yogurt, and almond milk.

4. If you prefer a sweeter taste, add honey to the mix.

5. Optional: Add a handful of ice cubes for a colder and thicker consistency.

6. Blend all the ingredients until smooth and well combined.

7. Taste the smoothie and adjust sweetness or thickness as desired by adding more honey or milk.

8. Pour the smoothie into a glass and enjoy the nutritious goodness of this spinach, banana, and chia seeds smoothie!

Greek yogurt parfait with granola and mixed berries

Ingredients:

- 1 cup Greek yogurt
- 1/2 cup granola
- 1 cup mixed berries (strawberries, blueberries, raspberries)
- 1 tablespoon honey (optional, for sweetness)

Instructions:

1. In a glass or a bowl, start with a layer of Greek yogurt at the bottom.
2. Add a layer of granola on top of the Greek yogurt.
3. Wash and prepare the mixed berries. Add a layer of mixed berries on top of the granola.
4. Repeat the layers until you reach the desired amount or the top of the container.
5. If you like, drizzle honey over the top for added sweetness.
6. Optionally, garnish with a few whole berries or a sprinkle of granola on top for texture.
7. Serve immediately and enjoy your delicious Greek yogurt parfait with granola and mixed berries!

Whole grain pancakes with sliced strawberries

Ingredients:

- 1 cup whole wheat flour
- 2 tablespoons sugar
- 1 teaspoon baking powder

- 1/2 teaspoon baking soda
- 1/4 teaspoon salt
- 1 cup buttermilk
- 1 large egg
- 2 tablespoons unsalted butter, melted
- 1 teaspoon vanilla extract
- Sliced strawberries for topping
- Maple syrup for serving

Instructions:

1. In a large bowl, whisk together the whole wheat flour, sugar, baking powder, baking soda, and salt.

2. In a separate bowl, whisk together the buttermilk, egg, melted butter, and vanilla extract.

3. Pour the wet ingredients into the dry ingredients and gently stir until just combined. Be careful not to overmix; a few lumps are okay.

4. Heat a griddle or non-stick skillet over medium heat and lightly grease with cooking spray or butter.

5. Pour 1/4 cup portions of batter onto the griddle for each pancake.

6. Cook until bubbles form on the surface of the pancake, then flip and cook the other side until golden brown.

7. Repeat until all the batter is used.

8. Serve the whole grain pancakes topped with sliced strawberries and drizzled with maple syrup.

Scrambled eggs with spinach and whole grain toast

Ingredients:

- 2 large eggs
- 1 cup fresh spinach leaves, washed and chopped
- Salt and pepper to taste
- 1 tablespoon olive oil or butter
- 2 slices of whole grain bread, toasted

Instructions:

1. Heat olive oil or butter in a non-stick skillet over medium heat.

2. Add the chopped spinach to the skillet and sauté until wilted, about 1-2 minutes.

3. In a bowl, whisk the eggs and season with salt and pepper.

4. Pour the whisked eggs into the skillet with the wilted spinach.

5. Gently scramble the eggs and spinach together until the eggs are cooked through but still moist.

6. Toast the whole grain bread slices.

7. Serve the scrambled eggs and spinach over the whole grain toast.

8. Optionally, season with additional salt and pepper to taste.

Overnight oats with almond milk, chia seeds, and sliced peaches

Ingredients:

- 1/2 cup rolled oats
- 1/2 cup almond milk
- 1 tablespoon chia seeds
- 1 ripe peach, sliced
- 1 tablespoon honey (optional, for sweetness)
- 1/4 teaspoon vanilla extract
- A pinch of salt

Instructions:

1. In a jar or container, combine rolled oats, almond milk, chia seeds, honey (if using), vanilla extract, and a pinch of salt.

2. Stir the ingredients well to ensure they are evenly mixed.

3. Add the sliced peaches on top of the oat mixture.

4. Seal the jar or container and refrigerate overnight, or for at least 4 hours.

5. The next morning, give the overnight oats a good stir.

6. If desired, add more almond milk to achieve your preferred consistency.

7. Top with additional peach slices and a drizzle of honey if you like.

8. Enjoy your delicious and nutritious overnight oats with almond milk, chia seeds, and sliced peaches!

Sweet Potato Hash

Ingredients:

- 2 medium-sized sweet potatoes, peeled and diced

- 1 red bell pepper, diced
- 1 yellow onion, finely chopped
- 2 cloves garlic, minced
- 2 tablespoons olive oil
- 1 teaspoon smoked paprika
- 1/2 teaspoon cumin
- Salt and pepper to taste
- Optional toppings: fried or poached eggs, avocado, green onions

Instructions:

1. In a large skillet, heat olive oil over medium heat.
2. Add the diced sweet potatoes and cook for about 8-10 minutes, stirring occasionally, until they begin to soften.
3. Add the chopped red bell pepper and onion to the skillet. Continue cooking for an additional 5-7 minutes, or until the vegetables are tender and slightly caramelized.
4. Stir in the minced garlic, smoked paprika, cumin, salt, and pepper. Cook for an additional 2-3 minutes to let the flavors meld.

5. Adjust seasoning to taste and continue cooking until the sweet potatoes are fully cooked and slightly crispy on the edges.

6. Optional: Top with fried or poached eggs, sliced avocado, or green onions for added flavor and texture.

7. Serve hot and enjoy your delicious sweet potato hash!

Avocado and tomato omelet with whole grain toast

Ingredients:

- 2 eggs
- 1/2 avocado, sliced
- 1/2 cup cherry tomatoes, halved
- Salt and pepper to taste
- 1 tablespoon olive oil
- 2 slices of whole grain bread, toasted

Instructions:

1. In a bowl, whisk the eggs and season with salt and pepper.

2. Heat olive oil in a non-stick skillet over medium heat.

3. Pour the whisked eggs into the skillet and let them set slightly.

4. Add sliced avocado and halved cherry tomatoes to one half of the omelet.

5. Once the eggs are mostly set, carefully fold the omelet in half over the filling.

6. Allow the omelet to cook until the eggs are fully set and the filling is warmed through.

7. Slide the omelet onto a plate.

8. Serve with toasted whole grain bread on the side.

Berry and kale smoothie with a scoop of protein powder

Ingredients:

- 1 cup mixed berries (strawberries, blueberries, raspberries)
- 1 cup chopped kale (stems removed)
- 1 banana
- 1 scoop of your favorite protein powder
- 1 cup almond milk (or any milk of your choice)
- Ice cubes (optional)

Instructions:

1. Place berries, chopped kale, banana, protein powder, and almond milk in a blender.
2. Blend until smooth and creamy.
3. Add ice cubes if you prefer a colder consistency.
4. Pour into a glass and enjoy your nutritious berry and kale smoothie with added protein!

Whole grain waffles with Greek yogurt and sliced banana

Ingredients:

- 1 cup whole wheat flour
- 1 tablespoon sugar
- 1 teaspoon baking powder
- 1/2 teaspoon baking soda
- 1/4 teaspoon salt
- 1 cup buttermilk
- 1 large egg
- 2 tablespoons melted butter
- 1 teaspoon vanilla extract
- Greek yogurt
- Sliced banana

Instructions:

1. In a large bowl, whisk together whole wheat flour, sugar, baking powder, baking soda, and salt.

2. In a separate bowl, whisk together buttermilk, egg, melted butter, and vanilla extract.

3. Pour the wet ingredients into the dry ingredients and stir until just combined.

4. Preheat your waffle iron and lightly grease it.

5. Pour the batter onto the waffle iron and cook according to the manufacturer's instructions until golden brown.

6. Once the waffles are cooked, spread Greek yogurt on top and add sliced bananas.

7. Serve warm and enjoy your wholesome whole grain waffles with Greek yogurt and sliced banana!

Chia seed pudding with mixed berries

Ingredients:

- 1/4 cup chia seeds
- 1 cup almond milk (or any milk of your choice)

- 1 tablespoon honey or maple syrup (adjust to taste)
- 1/2 teaspoon vanilla extract
- Mixed berries (strawberries, blueberries, raspberries)

Instructions:

1. In a bowl, combine chia seeds, almond milk, honey or maple syrup, and vanilla extract.
2. Stir the mixture well to ensure the chia seeds are evenly distributed.
3. Cover the bowl and refrigerate for at least 2 hours or overnight, allowing the chia seeds to absorb the liquid and create a pudding-like consistency.
4. Stir the chia pudding before serving to break up any clumps.
5. Wash and prepare the mixed berries.
6. Layer the chia seed pudding with mixed berries in serving glasses or bowls.
7. Optionally, drizzle with additional honey or maple syrup for sweetness.
8. Enjoy your nutritious and delicious chia seed pudding with mixed berries!

Whole grain English muffin with scrambled eggs and sliced avocado

Ingredients:

- 1 whole grain English muffin, split and toasted
- 2 eggs, scrambled
- 1/2 avocado, sliced
- Salt and pepper to taste
- Optional toppings: chopped herbs, hot sauce, or feta cheese

Instructions:

1. Toast the whole grain English muffin halves until golden brown.
2. In a bowl, scramble the eggs and season with salt and pepper.
3. Cook the scrambled eggs in a pan over medium heat until just set.
4. Place the scrambled eggs on one half of the toasted English muffin.
5. Top with sliced avocado.
6. Optional: Add additional toppings like chopped herbs, hot sauce, or crumbled feta cheese.
7. Place the other half of the English muffin on top to create a sandwich.

8. Serve immediately and enjoy your delicious whole grain English muffin with scrambled eggs and sliced avocado!

Banana and almond butter smoothie with a handful of spinach

Ingredients:
- 1 ripe banana
- 2 tablespoons almond butter
- Handful of fresh spinach leaves
- 1 cup almond milk (or any milk of your choice)
- Ice cubes (optional)

Instructions:
1. Peel the ripe banana and place it in a blender.
2. Add almond butter, fresh spinach leaves, and almond milk to the blender.
3. Optionally, add ice cubes for a colder and thicker consistency.
4. Blend until all ingredients are smooth and well combined.
5. Pour the smoothie into a glass and enjoy your nutritious banana and almond butter smoothie with a hint of spinach!

Whole grain bagel with smoked salmon, cream cheese, and capers

Ingredients:

- 1 whole grain bagel, sliced and toasted
- 2 oz smoked salmon
- 2 tablespoons cream cheese
- 1 tablespoon capers, drained
- Fresh dill for garnish
- Lemon wedges (optional)

Instructions:

1. Toast the sliced whole grain bagel until golden brown.
2. Spread a generous layer of cream cheese on each half of the bagel.
3. Lay smoked salmon on top of the cream cheese, evenly distributing it on both halves.
4. Sprinkle capers over the smoked salmon.
5. Garnish with fresh dill for added flavor.
6. Optionally, serve with lemon wedges on the side for a citrusy touch.
7. Put the two halves together to form a sandwich.

8. Enjoy your delightful whole grain bagel with smoked salmon, cream cheese, and capers!

Greek yogurt with sliced banana and a handful of walnuts

Ingredients:

- 1 cup Greek yogurt
- 1 ripe banana, sliced
- A handful of walnuts, chopped
- Honey or maple syrup (optional, for sweetness)

Instructions:

1. Spoon Greek yogurt into a bowl or serving dish.
2. Arrange sliced bananas on top of the yogurt.
3. Sprinkle chopped walnuts over the bananas and yogurt.
4. Optionally, drizzle honey or maple syrup for added sweetness.
5. Gently mix the ingredients together or enjoy in layers.
6. Serve immediately and savor your delicious and protein-packed Greek yogurt with sliced banana and walnuts!

Avocado and egg breakfast burrito with salsa on a whole wheat tortilla

Ingredients:

- 1 whole wheat tortilla
- 1 egg, scrambled
- 1/2 avocado, sliced
- Salsa (store-bought or homemade)
- Salt and pepper to taste
- Optional toppings: shredded cheese, chopped cilantro, or hot sauce

Instructions:

1. In a pan, scramble the egg until cooked through. Season with salt and pepper.
2. Warm the whole wheat tortilla in the pan or microwave for a few seconds.
3. Place the scrambled egg in the center of the tortilla.
4. Add sliced avocado on top of the eggs.
5. Spoon salsa over the avocado and egg mixture.
6. Optionally, add any additional toppings like shredded cheese, chopped cilantro, or hot sauce.

7. Fold the sides of the tortilla over the filling and roll it up to form a burrito.

8. Serve immediately and enjoy your delicious avocado and egg breakfast burrito with salsa!

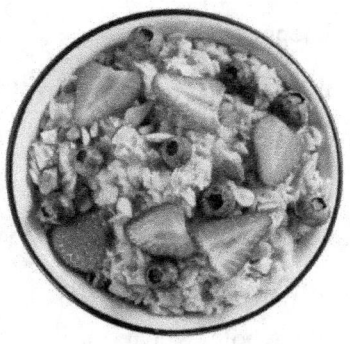

CHAPTER 4: LUNCH RECIPES

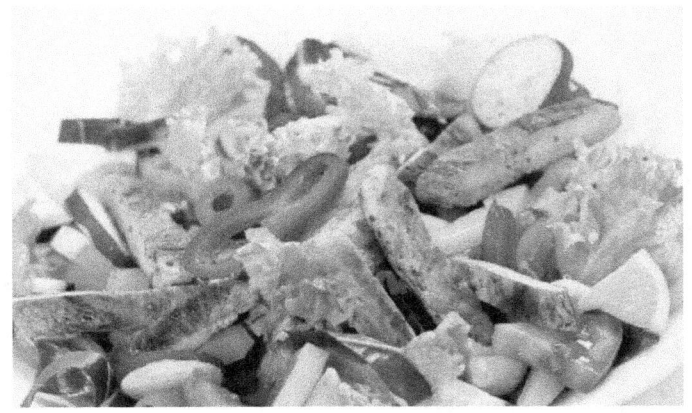

Grilled chicken salad with mixed greens and olive oil dressing

Ingredients:

For the Salad:

- Grilled chicken breast, sliced
- Mixed salad greens (e.g., spinach, arugula, romaine lettuce)
- Cherry tomatoes, halved
- Cucumber, sliced
- Red onion, thinly sliced
- Avocado, sliced (optional)
- Feta cheese, crumbled (optional)

For the Olive Oil Dressing:

- 3 tablespoons extra-virgin olive oil
- 1 tablespoon balsamic vinegar
- 1 teaspoon Dijon mustard
- 1 clove garlic, minced
- Salt and pepper to taste

Instructions:

1. In a large bowl, combine the mixed salad greens, cherry tomatoes, cucumber, red onion, and any optional ingredients like avocado or feta cheese.
2. Slice grilled chicken breast and arrange it on top of the salad.
3. In a small bowl, whisk together the olive oil, balsamic vinegar, Dijon mustard, minced garlic, salt, and pepper to make the dressing.
4. Drizzle the olive oil dressing over the salad and toss gently to coat the ingredients evenly.
5. Serve the grilled chicken salad immediately, and enjoy!

Lentil soup with a side of mixed vegetables

Lentil Soup:

Ingredients:

- 1 cup dried green or brown lentils, rinsed and drained
- 1 onion, finely chopped
- 2 carrots, diced
- 2 celery stalks, diced
- 3 cloves garlic, minced
- 1 can (14 oz) diced tomatoes
- 6 cups vegetable broth
- 1 teaspoon ground cumin
- 1 teaspoon ground coriander
- 1/2 teaspoon smoked paprika
- Salt and pepper to taste
- 2 tablespoons olive oil
- Fresh parsley for garnish (optional)
- Lemon wedges for serving (optional)

Instructions:

1. In a large pot, heat olive oil over medium heat. Add chopped onions, carrots, celery, and garlic. Sauté until the vegetables are softened.

2. Add cumin, coriander, smoked paprika, salt, and pepper. Stir well to coat the vegetables in the spices.

3. Pour in the vegetable broth, lentils, and diced tomatoes (with their juice). Bring the mixture to a boil.

4. Reduce the heat to low, cover the pot, and simmer for about 25-30 minutes or until the lentils are tender.

5. Adjust seasoning if needed and add more broth if you prefer a thinner soup.

6. Serve the lentil soup hot, garnished with fresh parsley and accompanied by lemon wedges on the side.

Mixed Vegetables:

Ingredients:

- 2 cups mixed vegetables (such as broccoli, cauliflower, carrots, and bell peppers)
- 1 tablespoon olive oil
- Salt and pepper to taste

- 1 teaspoon dried herbs (such as thyme or rosemary)

Instructions:

1. Preheat the oven to 400°F (200°C).
2. Toss the mixed vegetables with olive oil, salt, pepper, and dried herbs in a mixing bowl.
3. Spread the seasoned vegetables on a baking sheet in a single layer.
4. Roast in the preheated oven for about 20-25 minutes or until the vegetables are tender and lightly browned, stirring halfway through.
5. Serve the roasted mixed vegetables alongside the lentil soup.

Quinoa salad with cherry tomatoes, feta cheese, and olive oil

Ingredients:

- 1 cup quinoa, rinsed
- 2 cups water or vegetable broth
- 1 pint cherry tomatoes, halved
- 1/2 cup crumbled feta cheese
- 1/4 cup fresh parsley, chopped
- 1/4 cup Kalamata olives, pitted and sliced

- 3 tablespoons extra-virgin olive oil
- 2 tablespoons red wine vinegar
- Salt and pepper to taste
- Optional: 1/2 red onion, finely chopped

Instructions:

1. In a medium saucepan, combine quinoa and water (or vegetable broth). Bring to a boil, then reduce heat to low, cover, and simmer for 15-20 minutes, or until the quinoa is cooked and the liquid is absorbed. Fluff with a fork and let it cool.

2. In a large mixing bowl, combine the cooked quinoa, cherry tomatoes, feta cheese, fresh parsley, and Kalamata olives. If using red onion, add it at this point.

3. In a small bowl, whisk together the olive oil, red wine vinegar, salt, and pepper.

4. Pour the dressing over the quinoa mixture and toss gently to combine, ensuring everything is well coated.

5. Taste and adjust seasoning as needed.

6. Refrigerate the quinoa salad for at least 30 minutes before serving to allow the flavors to meld.

7. Before serving, give the salad a final toss and garnish with extra fresh parsley or crumbled feta if desired.

8. Serve chilled and enjoy your refreshing quinoa salad with cherry tomatoes, feta cheese, and olive oil! This salad can be a perfect side dish or a light and nutritious meal on its own.

Stir-fried tofu with broccoli and brown rice

Ingredients:

- 1 cup brown rice, cooked
- 1 block (14 oz) firm tofu, pressed and cubed
- 2 cups broccoli florets
- 2 tablespoons soy sauce
- 1 tablespoon sesame oil
- 1 tablespoon vegetable oil
- 1 tablespoon rice vinegar
- 1 tablespoon hoisin sauce
- 2 cloves garlic, minced
- 1 teaspoon ginger, grated
- Sesame seeds and green onions for garnish (optional)

Instructions:

1. Cook the brown rice according to package instructions and set aside.

2. Press the tofu to remove excess moisture, then cut it into cubes.

3. In a large pan or wok, heat vegetable oil over medium-high heat. Add tofu cubes and cook until golden brown on all sides.

4. Add minced garlic and grated ginger to the tofu, stirring for about 1 minute until fragrant.

5. Toss in broccoli florets and continue stir-frying for an additional 3-5 minutes until the broccoli is tender-crisp.

6. In a small bowl, mix together soy sauce, sesame oil, rice vinegar, and hoisin sauce. Pour the sauce over the tofu and broccoli, stirring to coat evenly.

7. Add the cooked brown rice to the pan, tossing everything together until well combined and heated through.

8. Garnish with sesame seeds and sliced green onions if desired.

9. Serve immediately and enjoy your delicious stir-fried tofu with broccoli and brown rice!

Chickpea salad with cherry tomatoes, cucumber, and lemon-tahini dressing

Ingredients:

- 1 can (15 oz) chickpeas, drained and rinsed
- 1 cup cherry tomatoes, halved
- 1 cucumber, diced
- 1/4 cup red onion, finely chopped
- 1/4 cup fresh parsley, chopped
- 2 tablespoons tahini
- 2 tablespoons fresh lemon juice
- 2 tablespoons olive oil
- 1 clove garlic, minced
- Salt and pepper to taste

Instructions:

1. In a large bowl, combine the chickpeas, cherry tomatoes, cucumber, red onion, and fresh parsley.
2. In a separate small bowl, whisk together the tahini, fresh lemon juice, olive oil, minced garlic, salt, and pepper until well combined.

3. Pour the lemon-tahini dressing over the chickpea mixture and toss until everything is evenly coated.

4. Adjust seasoning to taste, adding more salt, pepper, or lemon juice if needed.

5. Allow the salad to marinate for at least 15-20 minutes to let the flavors meld.

6. Serve chilled and enjoy this refreshing chickpea salad with cherry tomatoes, cucumber, and lemon-tahini dressing!

Turkey and vegetable wrap with whole wheat tortilla

Ingredients:

- 1 whole wheat tortilla
- 4-6 slices of turkey
- 1 cup shredded lettuce
- 1 medium tomato, thinly sliced
- 1/2 avocado, sliced
- 1/4 cucumber, thinly sliced
- 1/4 cup bell peppers, thinly sliced
- Your favorite light dressing

Instructions:

1. Lay the whole wheat tortilla flat on a clean surface.

2. Arrange the turkey slices evenly over the tortilla.

3. Add the shredded lettuce, sliced tomatoes, avocado, cucumber, and bell peppers on top of the turkey.

4. Drizzle your preferred light dressing over the veggies.

5. Carefully fold in the sides of the tortilla, then roll it up tightly from the bottom to create the wrap.

6. Slice the wrap in half diagonally for easier handling.

7. Serve and enjoy your wholesome turkey and vegetable wrap!

Quinoa-stuffed bell peppers with black beans and corn

Ingredients:

- 4 large bell peppers, halved and seeds removed
- 1 cup quinoa, rinsed
- 2 cups vegetable broth or water

- 1 can (15 oz) black beans, drained and rinsed
- 1 cup corn kernels (fresh or frozen)
- 1 cup diced tomatoes
- 1 cup shredded cheese (cheddar, Monterey Jack, or a Mexican blend)
- 1 teaspoon ground cumin
- 1 teaspoon chili powder
- 1/2 teaspoon garlic powder
- Salt and pepper to taste
- Olive oil for drizzling
- Fresh cilantro for garnish (optional)
- Avocado slices for serving (optional)
- Sour cream or Greek yogurt for serving (optional)

Instructions:

1. Preheat the oven to 375°F (190°C).
2. In a medium saucepan, combine quinoa and vegetable broth (or water). Bring to a boil, then reduce heat to low, cover, and simmer for 15-20 minutes or until the quinoa is cooked and the liquid is absorbed. Fluff with a fork and let it cool.

3. In a large mixing bowl, combine the cooked quinoa, black beans, corn, diced tomatoes, shredded cheese, ground cumin, chili powder, garlic powder, salt, and pepper. Mix well to combine.

4. Place the halved bell peppers in a baking dish. Stuff each pepper half with the quinoa mixture, pressing it down gently.

5. Drizzle a bit of olive oil over the stuffed peppers and cover the baking dish with aluminum foil.

6. Bake in the preheated oven for 25-30 minutes or until the peppers are tender.

7. Remove the foil and bake for an additional 5-10 minutes or until the cheese is melted and bubbly.

8. Remove from the oven and let it cool for a few minutes.

9. Garnish with fresh cilantro if desired.

10. Serve the quinoa-stuffed bell peppers with black beans and corn with optional avocado slices and a dollop of sour cream or Greek yogurt.

Spinach and feta stuffed chicken breast with quinoa

Ingredients:

For the Chicken:

- 4 boneless, skinless chicken breasts
- Salt and pepper, to taste
- 1 tablespoon olive oil

For the Spinach and Feta Stuffing:

- 2 cups fresh spinach, chopped
- 1/2 cup feta cheese, crumbled
- 2 cloves garlic, minced
- 1 tablespoon olive oil
- Salt and pepper, to taste

For the Quinoa:

- 1 cup quinoa, rinsed
- 2 cups chicken broth (or water)
- Salt, to taste

Instructions:

1. Preheat your oven to 375°F (190°C).
2. In a medium skillet, heat 1 tablespoon of olive oil over medium heat. Add minced garlic and sauté until fragrant.

3. Add chopped spinach to the skillet and cook until wilted. Season with salt and pepper to taste. Remove from heat and let it cool slightly.

4. In a bowl, combine the wilted spinach with crumbled feta cheese. Mix well to create the stuffing.

5. Make a pocket in each chicken breast by cutting a slit horizontally along the side, being careful not to cut all the way through.

6. Stuff each chicken breast with the spinach and feta mixture. Secure with toothpicks if needed.

7. Season the outside of the stuffed chicken breasts with salt and pepper.

8. In an oven-safe skillet, heat 1 tablespoon of olive oil over medium-high heat. Brown the stuffed chicken breasts on each side for about 2-3 minutes until golden brown.

9. Transfer the skillet to the preheated oven and bake for about 20-25 minutes or until the chicken is cooked through and reaches an internal temperature of 165°F (74°C).

10. While the chicken is baking, rinse the quinoa under cold water. In a saucepan, combine quinoa, chicken broth (or water), and a pinch of salt.

11. Bring to a boil, then reduce heat to low, cover, and simmer for about 15 minutes or until the quinoa is cooked and the liquid is absorbed.

12. Serve the spinach and feta stuffed chicken breast over a bed of quinoa. Enjoy your delicious and nutritious meal!

Lentil and vegetable curry with brown rice

Ingredients:

For the Lentil and Vegetable Curry:

- 1 cup dry lentils (red or green), rinsed and drained
- 1 large onion, finely chopped
- 3 cloves garlic, minced
- 1 tablespoon ginger, grated
- 1 bell pepper, diced
- 2 carrots, peeled and sliced
- 1 zucchini, diced

- 1 can (14 oz) diced tomatoes
- 1 can (14 oz) coconut milk
- 2 tablespoons curry powder
- 1 teaspoon ground cumin
- 1 teaspoon ground coriander
- 1/2 teaspoon turmeric
- 1/2 teaspoon cayenne pepper (adjust to taste for spiciness)
- Salt and pepper to taste
- 2 tablespoons vegetable oil
- Fresh cilantro for garnish

For the Brown Rice:

- 1 cup brown rice
- 2 cups water
- 1/2 teaspoon salt

Instructions:

1. Rinse the lentils under cold water and set aside.
2. In a large pot or Dutch oven, heat the vegetable oil over medium heat. Add chopped onions and sauté until they become translucent.
3. Add minced garlic and grated ginger to the pot. Sauté for an additional minute until fragrant.

4. Stir in curry powder, ground cumin, ground coriander, turmeric, and cayenne pepper. Mix well to coat the onions with the spices.

5. Add diced bell pepper, sliced carrots, and diced zucchini to the pot. Cook for a few minutes until the vegetables start to soften.

6. Pour in the diced tomatoes (with their juices), coconut milk, and rinsed lentils. Season with salt and pepper. Stir to combine.

7. Bring the mixture to a boil, then reduce the heat to low, cover, and simmer for about 20-25 minutes or until the lentils and vegetables are tender.

8. While the curry is simmering, rinse the brown rice under cold water. In a separate pot, combine the brown rice, water, and salt. Bring to a boil, then reduce the heat to low, cover, and simmer for about 45-50 minutes or until the rice is cooked and the water is absorbed.

9. Once the lentils and vegetables are cooked, taste and adjust the seasoning if needed.

10. Serve the lentil and vegetable curry over a bed of brown rice. Garnish with fresh cilantro.

Caprese salad with whole grain crackers

Ingredients:

- 2 large tomatoes, sliced
- 1 ball of fresh mozzarella cheese, sliced
- Fresh basil leaves
- Extra virgin olive oil
- Balsamic glaze
- Salt and pepper to taste
- Whole grain crackers

Instructions:

1. Arrange the tomato and mozzarella slices alternately on a serving platter.
2. Tuck fresh basil leaves between the tomato and mozzarella slices.
3. Drizzle extra virgin olive oil over the salad.
4. Season with salt and pepper to taste.
5. Just before serving, drizzle balsamic glaze over the salad for a sweet and tangy flavor.
6. Serve the Caprese salad with a side of whole grain crackers.

Chickpea and vegetable wrap with a side of mixed greens

Chickpea and Vegetable Wrap:

Ingredients:

- 1 can (15 oz) chickpeas, drained and rinsed
- 1 tablespoon olive oil
- 1 teaspoon ground cumin
- 1 teaspoon smoked paprika
- Salt and pepper to taste
- 4 whole-grain or spinach wraps
- 1 cup hummus
- 1 cucumber, thinly sliced
- 1 bell pepper (any color), thinly sliced
- 1 large carrot, grated
- 1 cup cherry tomatoes, halved
- Fresh cilantro or parsley for garnish (optional)

Instructions:

1. In a medium-sized bowl, toss the chickpeas with olive oil, cumin, smoked paprika, salt, and pepper until well-coated.

2. Heat a skillet over medium heat. Add the seasoned chickpeas and cook for 5-7 minutes, stirring occasionally, until they are golden brown and crispy. Remove from heat.

3. Warm the wraps according to package instructions.

4. Assemble the wraps by spreading a generous layer of hummus on each wrap. Top with the crispy chickpeas, cucumber slices, bell pepper slices, grated carrot, and cherry tomatoes.

5. Garnish with fresh cilantro or parsley if desired.

6. Roll up the wraps tightly, folding in the sides as you go.

Mixed Greens Salad:

Ingredients:

- 4 cups mixed salad greens (such as spinach, arugula, and romaine)
- 1 cup cherry tomatoes, halved
- 1/2 cucumber, sliced
- 1/4 red onion, thinly sliced
- 2 tablespoons balsamic vinaigrette dressing

Instructions:

1. In a large bowl, combine the mixed salad greens, cherry tomatoes, cucumber, and red onion.

2. Drizzle the balsamic vinaigrette dressing over the salad and toss gently to coat.

3. Serve the Chickpea and Vegetable Wraps with a side of Mixed Greens for a delicious and healthy meal.

Mediterranean-style grilled chicken salad with olives and feta

Ingredients:

For the Grilled Chicken:

- 4 boneless, skinless chicken breasts
- 2 tablespoons olive oil
- 2 cloves garlic, minced
- 1 teaspoon dried oregano
- 1 teaspoon dried thyme
- Salt and pepper to taste
- Juice of 1 lemon

For the Salad:

- 6 cups mixed salad greens (romaine, arugula, spinach, etc.)

- 1 cup cherry tomatoes, halved
- 1 cucumber, sliced
- 1/2 red onion, thinly sliced
- 1/2 cup Kalamata olives, pitted and halved
- 1/2 cup crumbled feta cheese

For the Dressing:

- 1/4 cup extra-virgin olive oil
- 2 tablespoons red wine vinegar
- 1 teaspoon Dijon mustard
- 1 teaspoon honey
- Salt and pepper to taste

Instructions:

For the Grilled Chicken:

1. In a bowl, mix together olive oil, minced garlic, dried oregano, dried thyme, salt, pepper, and lemon juice to create the marinade.
2. Place the chicken breasts in a resealable plastic bag or shallow dish. Pour the marinade over the chicken, ensuring it's well-coated. Marinate for at least 30 minutes, or ideally, let it marinate in the refrigerator for a few hours.

3. Preheat the grill to medium-high heat. Grill the chicken for about 6-8 minutes per side or until fully cooked and have nice grill marks. Allow the chicken to rest for a few minutes before slicing it into strips.

For the Salad:

1. In a large salad bowl, combine the mixed greens, cherry tomatoes, cucumber, red onion, Kalamata olives, and crumbled feta cheese.

For the Dressing:

1. In a small bowl, whisk together the extra-virgin olive oil, red wine vinegar, Dijon mustard, honey, salt, and pepper until well combined.

2. Pour the dressing over the salad and toss gently to coat.

Assembly:

1. Arrange the grilled chicken strips on top of the salad.

2. Serve immediately, and enjoy your Mediterranean-style Grilled Chicken Salad with Olives and Feta!

Quinoa and black bean bowl with avocado and salsa

Ingredients:

For the Quinoa and Black Bean Mixture:

- 1 cup quinoa, rinsed

- 2 cups vegetable broth or water

- 1 can (15 oz) black beans, drained and rinsed

- 1 teaspoon ground cumin

- 1 teaspoon chili powder

- Salt and pepper to taste

- Juice of 1 lime

For the Avocado and Salsa Topping:

- 2 ripe avocados, diced

- 1 cup cherry tomatoes, diced

- 1/2 red onion, finely chopped

- 1/4 cup fresh cilantro, chopped

- Juice of 1 lime

- Salt and pepper to taste

Instructions:

For the Quinoa and Black Bean Mixture:

1. In a medium saucepan, combine quinoa and vegetable broth (or water).

2. Bring to a boil, then reduce heat to low, cover, and simmer for 15-20 minutes, or until quinoa is cooked and water is absorbed.

3. In a separate pan, heat black beans over medium heat. Add ground cumin, chili powder, salt, and pepper. Cook for 5-7 minutes, stirring occasionally. Once heated through, add the lime juice and stir to combine.

4. Combine the cooked quinoa and black bean mixture. Adjust seasoning if needed.

For the Avocado and Salsa Topping:

1. In a bowl, gently combine diced avocados, cherry tomatoes, red onion, and fresh cilantro.

2. Squeeze lime juice over the mixture and season with salt and pepper. Toss gently to combine.

Assembly:

1. Spoon the quinoa and black bean mixture into bowls.

2. Top each bowl with the avocado and salsa mixture.

3. Optionally, garnish with extra cilantro and a lime wedge.

4. Serve immediately and enjoy your delicious Quinoa and Black Bean Bowl with Avocado and Salsa!

Spinach and mushroom omelet with a side of whole grain toast

Spinach and Mushroom Omelet:

Ingredients:

- 3 large eggs
- 1/4 cup milk (or a dairy-free alternative)
- Salt and pepper to taste
- 1 tablespoon olive oil
- 1 cup baby spinach, chopped
- 1/2 cup mushrooms, sliced
- 1/4 cup red bell pepper, diced
- 1/4 cup feta cheese, crumbled (optional)
- Fresh herbs (such as parsley or chives) for garnish (optional)

Instructions:

1. In a bowl, whisk together the eggs, milk, salt, and pepper until well combined.
2. Heat olive oil in a non-stick skillet over medium heat.

3. Add mushrooms and red bell pepper to the skillet. Sauté for 2-3 minutes until they begin to soften.

4. Add the chopped spinach to the skillet and continue to sauté for an additional 2-3 minutes until the spinach is wilted.

5. Pour the whisked egg mixture over the vegetables in the skillet.

6. Allow the eggs to set around the edges. As the eggs set, gently lift the edges with a spatula, tilting the skillet to let the uncooked eggs flow to the edges.

7. Once the omelet is mostly set but still slightly runny on top, sprinkle crumbled feta cheese over one half of the omelet.

8. Carefully fold the other half of the omelet over the cheese.

9. Cook for an additional 1-2 minutes until the cheese is melted, and the omelet is cooked through.

10. Slide the omelet onto a plate and garnish with fresh herbs if desired.

Whole Grain Toast:

- Toast slices of your favorite whole grain bread.

Assembly:

1. Serve the Spinach and Mushroom Omelet on a plate.
2. Place the whole grain toast slices on the side.
3. Optionally, garnish the omelet with additional fresh herbs.
4. Enjoy your nutritious and flavorful Spinach and Mushroom Omelet with a side of Whole Grain Toast!

Lentil and vegetable soup with a whole grain roll

Lentil and Vegetable Soup:

Ingredients:

- 1 cup dried green or brown lentils, rinsed and drained
- 1 tablespoon olive oil
- 1 onion, diced
- 2 carrots, diced
- 2 celery stalks, diced
- 3 cloves garlic, minced
- 1 teaspoon ground cumin
- 1 teaspoon ground coriander

- 1 teaspoon smoked paprika

- 1 can (14 oz) diced tomatoes

- 6 cups vegetable broth

- 2 bay leaves

- Salt and pepper to taste

- 3 cups chopped mixed vegetables (e.g., zucchini, bell peppers, spinach, kale)

- Fresh parsley for garnish

Instructions:

1. In a large pot, heat olive oil over medium heat. Add the diced onion, carrots, and celery. Sauté for 5-7 minutes until the vegetables are softened.

2. Add minced garlic, ground cumin, ground coriander, and smoked paprika. Cook for an additional 1-2 minutes until the spices are fragrant.

3. Add lentils, diced tomatoes, vegetable broth, bay leaves, salt, and pepper to the pot. Bring to a boil, then reduce the heat to simmer. Cover and let it simmer for about 25-30 minutes, or until lentils are tender.

4. Add the chopped mixed vegetables and cook for an additional 10-15 minutes until all the vegetables are tender.

5. Adjust seasoning to taste and remove the bay leaves.

6. Ladle the soup into bowls, garnish with fresh parsley, and serve hot.

Whole Grain Roll:

- Purchase or bake whole grain rolls according to package instructions.

Assembly:

1. Serve a generous portion of Lentil and Vegetable Soup in a bowl.

2. Place a whole grain roll on the side.

3. Optionally, garnish the soup with additional fresh herbs.

4. Enjoy your comforting and nutritious Lentil and Vegetable Soup with a side of Whole Grain Roll!

Turkey and vegetable stir-fry with brown rice

Ingredients:

For the Stir-Fry:

- 1 lb ground turkey
- 2 tablespoons soy sauce (low-sodium)
- 1 tablespoon oyster sauce
- 1 tablespoon hoisin sauce
- 1 tablespoon sesame oil
- 1 tablespoon vegetable oil
- 3 cloves garlic, minced
- 1 tablespoon ginger, grated
- 1 red bell pepper, thinly sliced
- 1 yellow bell pepper, thinly sliced
- 1 cup broccoli florets
- 1 carrot, julienned
- 1 cup snap peas, ends trimmed
- 4 green onions, sliced
- Sesame seeds for garnish (optional)

For the Brown Rice:

- 1 cup brown rice
- 2 cups water

- 1/2 teaspoon salt

Instructions:

For the Brown Rice:

1. Rinse the brown rice under cold water.

2. In a medium saucepan, combine the rinsed brown rice, water, and salt. Bring to a boil.

3. Reduce heat to low, cover, and simmer for 45-50 minutes or until the rice is tender and water is absorbed. Fluff the rice with a fork.

For the Turkey and Vegetable Stir-Fry:

1. In a small bowl, mix together soy sauce, oyster sauce, and hoisin sauce. Set aside.

2. In a large wok or skillet, heat sesame oil and vegetable oil over medium-high heat.

3. Add minced garlic and grated ginger, and sauté for 1-2 minutes until fragrant.

4. Add ground turkey to the wok. Cook until browned and fully cooked, breaking it apart with a spatula as it cooks.

5. Add the bell peppers, broccoli, carrot, and snap peas to the wok. Stir-fry for 4-5 minutes until the vegetables are tender-crisp.

6. Pour the sauce over the turkey and vegetables. Toss everything together until well coated and heated through.

7. Stir in sliced green onions and cook for an additional 1-2 minutes.

Assembly:

1. Serve the Turkey and Vegetable Stir-Fry over a bed of brown rice.

2. Garnish with sesame seeds if desired.

3. Enjoy your delicious and nutritious Turkey and Vegetable Stir-Fry with Brown Rice!

Chickpea and vegetable curry with quinoa

Ingredients:

For the Chickpea and Vegetable Curry:

- 2 tablespoons coconut oil
- 1 large onion, finely chopped
- 3 cloves garlic, minced
- 1 tablespoon ginger, grated
- 1 can (15 oz) chickpeas, drained and rinsed
- 1 large sweet potato, peeled and diced
- 1 red bell pepper, diced

- 1 zucchini, diced
- 1 cup cherry tomatoes, halved
- 1 can (14 oz) coconut milk
- 2 tablespoons tomato paste
- 2 tablespoons curry powder
- 1 teaspoon ground turmeric
- 1 teaspoon ground cumin
- 1/2 teaspoon cayenne pepper (optional, for heat)
- Salt and pepper to taste
- Fresh cilantro for garnish

For the Quinoa:

- 1 cup quinoa, rinsed
- 2 cups vegetable broth or water
- Salt to taste

Instructions:

For the Quinoa:

1. Rinse the quinoa under cold water.
2. In a saucepan, combine quinoa, vegetable broth (or water), and a pinch of salt. Bring to a boil.
3. Reduce heat to low, cover, and simmer for 15-20 minutes, or until quinoa is cooked and water is absorbed. Fluff the quinoa with a fork.

For the Chickpea and Vegetable Curry:

1. In a large skillet or pot, heat coconut oil over medium heat.

2. Add chopped onion, garlic, and grated ginger. Sauté for 2-3 minutes until the onions are softened and fragrant.

3. Add curry powder, ground turmeric, ground cumin, and cayenne pepper (if using). Stir well to coat the onions in the spices.

4. Add diced sweet potato, red bell pepper, zucchini, and cherry tomatoes to the pot. Cook for 5-7 minutes until the vegetables start to soften.

5. Pour in the coconut milk and add tomato paste. Stir to combine.

6. Add chickpeas to the pot. Season with salt and pepper to taste. Stir well, cover, and let it simmer for 15-20 minutes, or until the sweet potatoes are tender.

7. Adjust seasoning if needed and let the curry simmer for an additional 5 minutes.

Assembly:

1. Serve the Chickpea and Vegetable Curry over a bed of cooked quinoa.

2. Garnish with fresh cilantro.

3. Enjoy your flavorful and nutritious Chickpea and Vegetable Curry with Quinoa!

Shrimp and vegetable kebabs with whole grain couscous

Shrimp and Vegetable Kebabs:

Ingredients:

- 1 pound large shrimp, peeled and deveined
- 1 zucchini, sliced into rounds
- 1 bell pepper (any color), cut into chunks
- 1 red onion, cut into chunks
- Cherry tomatoes
- 2 tablespoons olive oil
- 2 cloves garlic, minced
- 1 teaspoon lemon zest
- 1 tablespoon lemon juice
- 1 teaspoon dried oregano
- Salt and pepper to taste
- Wooden skewers, soaked in water for 30 minutes

Instructions:

1. In a bowl, whisk together olive oil, minced garlic, lemon zest, lemon juice, dried oregano, salt, and pepper to create the marinade.

2. Thread shrimp, zucchini slices, bell pepper chunks, red onion chunks, and cherry tomatoes onto the soaked skewers, alternating the ingredients.

3. Place the skewers in a shallow dish and brush them with the marinade, ensuring they are well-coated. Let them marinate for at least 15-20 minutes.

4. Preheat the grill or grill pan over medium-high heat.

5. Grill the shrimp and vegetable kebabs for 3-4 minutes per side, or until the shrimp are opaque and the vegetables are slightly charred.

6. Remove the kebabs from the grill and let them rest for a few minutes.

Whole Grain Couscous:

Ingredients:

- 1 cup whole grain couscous
- 1 1/4 cups vegetable broth or water
- 1 tablespoon olive oil

- Salt and pepper to taste

Instructions:

1. In a saucepan, bring vegetable broth (or water) and olive oil to a boil.

2. Stir in whole grain couscous, cover the pot, and remove it from the heat. Let it sit for 5 minutes.

3. Fluff the couscous with a fork and season with salt and pepper to taste.

Assembly:

1. Serve the Shrimp and Vegetable Kebabs over a bed of whole grain couscous.

2. Optionally, garnish with fresh herbs like parsley or cilantro.

3. Enjoy your flavorful and nutritious Shrimp and Vegetable Kebabs with Whole Grain Couscous!

"I honor my body with nutrient-rich foods that promote healing."

"Each day, I am making positive changes for my liver's well-being."

CHAPTER 5: SNACK RECIPES

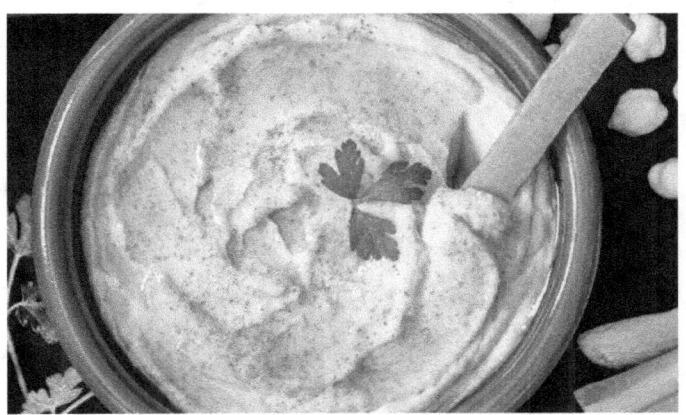

Greek yogurt with sliced cucumber

Ingredients:

- 1 cup Greek yogurt
- 1 medium cucumber, thinly sliced
- 1 tablespoon extra virgin olive oil
- 1 tablespoon fresh dill, chopped
- 1 clove garlic, minced (optional)
- Salt and pepper to taste

Instructions:

1. Wash and thinly slice the cucumber.
2. In a bowl, combine Greek yogurt, sliced cucumber, and chopped fresh dill.

3. If you like, add minced garlic for extra flavor. You can also adjust the quantity based on your preference.

4. Drizzle extra virgin olive oil over the mixture and gently toss everything together.

5. Season with salt and pepper to taste. Be mindful of the salt, as feta cheese (if added later) can also contribute to the overall saltiness.

6. Allow the flavors to meld by refrigerating for at least 15-20 minutes before serving.

7. Optionally, you can add some crumbled feta cheese on top before serving for an extra layer of flavor.

Apple slices with almond butter

Ingredients:

- 2 medium-sized apples (e.g., Honeycrisp, Gala, or Fuji)
- 1/2 cup almond butter
- 2 tablespoons honey or maple syrup (optional, for drizzling)
- 2 tablespoons chopped almonds (optional, for garnish)

- Cinnamon powder (optional, for sprinkling)

Instructions:

1. Wash and core the apples. Slice them into thin rounds or wedges. If you prefer, you can leave the skin on for added texture and nutrients.

2. In a small microwave-safe bowl, gently heat the almond butter for about 20-30 seconds until it becomes slightly more fluid. Alternatively, you can warm it on the stovetop using low heat.

3. Arrange the apple slices on a serving plate or platter.

4. Using a butter knife or a small spoon, spread a generous amount of almond butter onto each apple slice.

5. If desired, drizzle honey or maple syrup over the almond butter for a touch of sweetness.

6. Optional: Sprinkle chopped almonds on top for added crunch and texture.

7. If you enjoy the flavor of cinnamon, dust a little cinnamon powder over the apple slices.

8. Serve immediately and enjoy your delicious and nutritious apple slices with almond butter!

Carrot and celery sticks with hummus

Ingredients:

- 4 medium-sized carrots, peeled and cut into sticks
- 4 celery stalks, washed and cut into sticks
- 1 cup hummus (store-bought or homemade)
- Olive oil (optional, for drizzling)
- Paprika or smoked paprika (optional, for sprinkling)
- Fresh parsley, chopped (optional, for garnish)

Instructions:

1. Wash, peel, and cut the carrots and celery into sticks.
2. Arrange the carrot and celery sticks on a serving platter.
3. Place the hummus in a bowl or a small serving dish.
4. Optionally, drizzle a bit of olive oil over the hummus for extra richness.
5. Sprinkle a pinch of paprika or smoked paprika on top of the hummus for added flavor and a pop of color.

6. Garnish with fresh chopped parsley for a burst of freshness.

7. Serve the carrot and celery sticks alongside the hummus, creating a visually appealing and nutritious snack.

8. Dip the carrot and celery sticks into the hummus and enjoy!

Cottage cheese with pineapple chunks

Ingredients:

- 1 cup cottage cheese (low-fat or regular)
- 1 cup fresh pineapple chunks (or canned pineapple chunks, drained)
- 1 tablespoon honey (optional, for drizzling)
- Mint leaves (optional, for garnish)

Instructions:

1. In a bowl, scoop out the desired amount of cottage cheese.

2. Add fresh pineapple chunks to the cottage cheese. If using canned pineapple chunks, make sure to drain them well before adding.

3. Gently toss the cottage cheese and pineapple together until well combined.

4. Optional: Drizzle honey over the cottage cheese and pineapple for a touch of sweetness. Adjust the amount of honey based on your preference.

5. Garnish with fresh mint leaves for a burst of freshness and added aroma.

6. Serve immediately and enjoy this simple and nutritious cottage cheese with pineapple!

Mixed nuts and dried fruits

Ingredients:

- 1 cup mixed nuts (almonds, walnuts, cashews, pecans, etc.)
- 1/2 cup dried fruits (apricots, raisins, cranberries, figs, dates, etc.)
- 1 tablespoon honey or maple syrup
- 1/2 teaspoon cinnamon (optional)
- Pinch of salt

Instructions:

1. Preheat your oven to 325°F (163°C).

2. In a bowl, combine the mixed nuts and dried fruits.

3. Drizzle honey or maple syrup over the mixture and toss to coat evenly.

4. If desired, sprinkle cinnamon over the nuts and fruits for added flavor.

5. Spread the mixture evenly on a baking sheet lined with parchment paper.

6. Sprinkle a pinch of salt over the mixture for a sweet and salty balance.

7. Bake in the preheated oven for about 10-15 minutes, stirring halfway through to ensure even toasting.

8. Keep a close eye on the nuts to prevent burning; they should be golden brown and fragrant when done.

9. Remove from the oven and let the mixed nuts and dried fruits cool completely.

10. Once cooled, break up any clusters and transfer the mixture to an airtight container for storage.

11. Enjoy the mixed nuts and dried fruits as a snack, topping for yogurt or oatmeal, or as a trail mix.

Baked Sweet Potato Chips

Ingredients:

- 2 medium sweet potatoes, washed and peeled
- 2 tablespoons olive oil

- 1 teaspoon paprika
- 1/2 teaspoon garlic powder
- 1/2 teaspoon salt (adjust to taste)
- 1/4 teaspoon black pepper
- Optional: cayenne pepper for a bit of heat

Instructions:

1. Preheat your oven to 375°F (190°C). Line two baking sheets with parchment paper.

2. Using a mandoline slicer or a sharp knife, thinly slice the sweet potatoes into rounds. Aim for uniform thickness to ensure even baking.

3. In a large bowl, toss the sweet potato slices with olive oil, paprika, garlic powder, salt, pepper, and cayenne pepper if using. Make sure the slices are well coated.

4. Arrange the sweet potato slices in a single layer on the prepared baking sheets, ensuring they don't overlap.

5. Bake in the preheated oven for 15-20 minutes, flipping the slices halfway through, until the edges are golden brown and the chips are crisp.

6. Keep an eye on the chips towards the end of the baking time to prevent burning.

7. Once done, remove from the oven and let the sweet potato chips cool on the baking sheets for a few minutes. They will continue to crisp up as they cool.

8. Transfer the chips to a wire rack to cool completely.

9. Serve the baked sweet potato chips as a healthy snack or side dish.

Edamame beans with a sprinkle of sea salt

Ingredients:

- 2 cups edamame beans (fresh or frozen)
- Sea salt, to taste

Instructions:

1. If using frozen edamame, thaw them according to the package instructions.

2. Bring a pot of water to a boil and add a pinch of salt.

3. Add the edamame beans to the boiling water and cook for about 3-5 minutes, or until they are heated through.

4. Drain the edamame and transfer them to a serving bowl.

5. While the edamame are still warm, sprinkle sea salt over them. Start with a small amount and add more to taste.

6. Toss the edamame gently to ensure the salt is evenly distributed.

7. Serve the edamame beans as a snack, appetizer, or side dish.

8. Enjoy your simple and nutritious edamame beans with a sprinkle of sea salt!

Sliced bell peppers with guacamole

Ingredients:

For Guacamole:

- 2 ripe avocados, peeled and pitted
- 1 small red onion, finely diced
- 1-2 tomatoes, diced
- 1-2 cloves garlic, minced
- 1 lime, juiced
- Salt and pepper to taste
- Optional: cilantro, diced jalapeño for added flavor and heat

For Sliced Bell Peppers:

- Assorted bell peppers (red, yellow, green), sliced

Instructions:

For Guacamole:

1. In a bowl, mash the ripe avocados using a fork or potato masher.

2. Add diced red onion, diced tomatoes, minced garlic, lime juice, salt, and pepper to the mashed avocados.

3. Optional: Add chopped cilantro and diced jalapeño for extra flavor. Adjust the quantities based on your taste preferences.

4. Mix all the ingredients together until well combined.

5. Taste the guacamole and adjust the seasonings if needed. You can add more lime juice, salt, or pepper according to your liking.

6. Cover the guacamole with plastic wrap, ensuring it directly touches the surface of the guacamole to prevent browning. Refrigerate until ready to serve.

For Sliced Bell Peppers:

1. Wash and slice the bell peppers into strips or rings.

2. Arrange the sliced bell peppers on a serving platter.

3. Spoon the guacamole into a serving bowl and place it in the center of the sliced bell peppers.

4. Optionally, garnish the guacamole with additional cilantro or a lime wedge.

5. Serve the sliced bell peppers with guacamole as a colorful and flavorful snack or appetizer.

Handful of cherry tomatoes with mozzarella cheese

Ingredients:

- Cherry tomatoes
- Fresh mozzarella cheese balls (bocconcini)
- Fresh basil leaves (optional)
- Extra-virgin olive oil
- Balsamic glaze (optional)
- Salt and pepper to taste

Instructions:

1. Wash the cherry tomatoes and cut them in half. If you prefer, you can leave them whole.

2. Drain the mozzarella cheese balls if they are in liquid. You can also use mini mozzarella balls or cut larger mozzarella into bite-sized pieces.

3. On a serving platter or individual plates, arrange the cherry tomato halves and mozzarella cheese.

4. If using, add fresh basil leaves to the platter for added flavor and freshness.

5. Drizzle extra-virgin olive oil over the tomatoes and mozzarella. You can be generous with the olive oil as it adds richness to the dish.

6. Optionally, add a few drops of balsamic glaze for a sweet and tangy touch.

7. Sprinkle salt and pepper over the tomatoes and mozzarella to taste. You can also add a pinch of dried oregano if you like.

8. Gently toss the ingredients together or serve them as a beautiful, layered arrangement.

9. Serve immediately as a refreshing snack or appetizer.

Mixed nuts and dried cranberries

Ingredients:

- 1 cup mixed nuts (almonds, walnuts, cashews, pistachios, etc.)
- 1/2 cup dried cranberries

Instructions:

1. In a bowl, combine the mixed nuts and dried cranberries.
2. Toss the mixture together until the nuts and cranberries are evenly distributed.
3. Adjust the ratio of nuts to cranberries based on your preference.
4. Your mixed nuts and dried cranberries snack is ready to be enjoyed!

Sliced cucumber with tzatziki sauce

Ingredients:

For Tzatziki Sauce:

- 1 cup Greek yogurt
- 1 cucumber, finely grated
- 2 cloves garlic, minced
- 1 tablespoon fresh dill, chopped

- 1 tablespoon fresh mint, chopped
- 1 tablespoon extra-virgin olive oil
- 1 teaspoon lemon juice
- Salt and pepper to taste

For Sliced Cucumber:

- Cucumbers, washed and sliced

Instructions:

For Tzatziki Sauce:

1. In a bowl, combine Greek yogurt, finely grated cucumber, minced garlic, chopped dill, chopped mint, extra-virgin olive oil, lemon juice, salt, and pepper.
2. Mix all the ingredients until well combined.
3. Taste the tzatziki sauce and adjust the seasonings according to your liking.
4. Refrigerate the tzatziki sauce for at least 30 minutes to allow the flavors to meld.

For Sliced Cucumber with Tzatziki Sauce:

1. Wash and slice the cucumbers into rounds.
2. Arrange the cucumber slices on a serving platter.
3. Stir the tzatziki sauce to ensure it's well mixed.
4. Spoon the tzatziki sauce onto each cucumber slice.

5. Optionally, garnish with additional fresh herbs or a drizzle of olive oil.

6. Serve immediately and enjoy your refreshing snack of sliced cucumber with tzatziki sauce!

Sliced mango with a squeeze of lime

Ingredients:
- Ripe mangoes, peeled and sliced
- Fresh lime

Instructions:
1. Peel the mangoes and cut them into slices. You can use the "cheek" of the mango by slicing along either side of the pit.

2. Arrange the mango slices on a serving plate or platter.

3. Cut the lime in half.

4. Squeeze fresh lime juice over the sliced mango. The lime juice enhances the sweetness of the mango and adds a citrusy kick.

5. Optionally, you can zest a bit of lime peel over the mango slices for added flavor.

6. Serve the sliced mango with lime immediately for a refreshing and tropical snack.

Mixed nuts and dried apricots

Ingredients:

- 1 cup mixed nuts (almonds, walnuts, cashews, pistachios, etc.)
- 1/2 cup dried apricots, chopped

Instructions:

1. In a bowl, combine the mixed nuts and dried apricots.
2. Toss the mixture together until the nuts and apricots are evenly distributed.
3. Adjust the ratio of nuts to apricots based on your preference.
4. Your mixed nuts and dried apricots snack is ready to be enjoyed!

Brown Rice Cakes with Guacamole

Ingredients:

For Guacamole:

- 2 ripe avocados, peeled and pitted
- 1 small red onion, finely diced
- 1-2 tomatoes, diced
- 1-2 cloves garlic, minced

- 1 lime, juiced
- Salt and pepper to taste
- Optional: cilantro, diced jalapeño for added flavor and heat

For Brown Rice Cakes:

- Brown rice cakes
- Olive oil (for brushing, optional)
- Salt and pepper to taste

Instructions:

For Guacamole:

1. In a bowl, mash the ripe avocados using a fork or potato masher.
2. Add diced red onion, diced tomatoes, minced garlic, lime juice, salt, and pepper to the mashed avocados.
3. Optional: Add chopped cilantro and diced jalapeño for extra flavor. Adjust the quantities based on your taste preferences.
4. Mix all the ingredients together until well combined.
5. Taste the guacamole and adjust the seasonings if needed. You can add more lime juice, salt, or pepper according to your liking.

6. Cover the guacamole with plastic wrap, ensuring it directly touches the surface of the guacamole to prevent browning. Refrigerate until ready to serve.

For Brown Rice Cakes:

1. If desired, lightly brush the brown rice cakes with olive oil for added flavor and a slightly crispy texture.
2. Place the brown rice cakes on a serving platter.
3. Season the rice cakes with a sprinkle of salt and pepper.

Assembly:

1. Spoon a generous amount of guacamole onto each brown rice cake.
2. Optionally, garnish with additional cilantro or a squeeze of lime juice.
3. Serve immediately and enjoy your delicious Brown Rice Cakes with Guacamole!

"I am resilient, and my body is capable of positive transformation."

"I choose foods that love my liver and support its optimal function."

CHAPTER 6: DINNER RECIPES

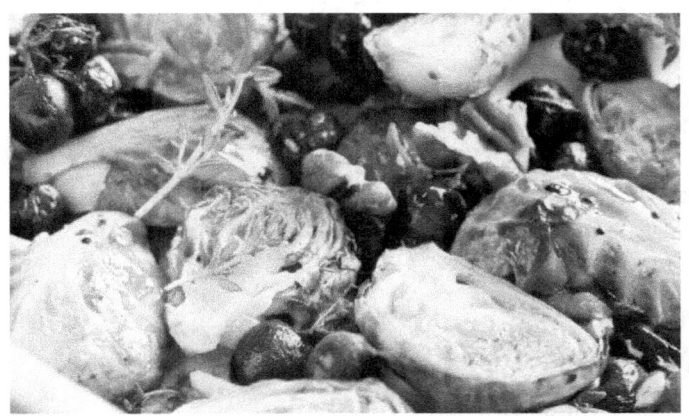

Quinoa-stuffed acorn squash with roasted Brussels sprouts

Ingredients:

For Quinoa-Stuffed Acorn Squash:

- 2 acorn squashes, halved and seeds removed
- 1 cup quinoa, rinsed
- 2 cups vegetable broth or water
- 1 tablespoon olive oil
- 1 onion, finely chopped
- 2 cloves garlic, minced
- 1 teaspoon ground cumin
- 1 teaspoon paprika

- Salt and pepper to taste
- 1/2 cup dried cranberries or raisins
- 1/2 cup chopped pecans or walnuts
- Fresh parsley or cilantro for garnish

For Roasted Brussels Sprouts:

- 2 cups Brussels sprouts, trimmed and halved
- 2 tablespoons olive oil
- Salt and pepper to taste

Instructions:

For Quinoa-Stuffed Acorn Squash:

1. Preheat the oven to 375°F (190°C).

2. Place the acorn squash halves, cut side up, on a baking sheet. Drizzle with olive oil, and season with salt and pepper.

3. Roast the acorn squash in the preheated oven for 30-40 minutes or until the squash is tender when pierced with a fork.

4. While the squash is roasting, rinse the quinoa under cold water. In a medium saucepan, combine quinoa and vegetable broth or water. Bring to a boil, then reduce the heat, cover, and simmer for 15-20 minutes, or until the quinoa is cooked and liquid is absorbed.

5. In a skillet, heat olive oil over medium heat. Add chopped onion and cook until translucent.

6. Add minced garlic, ground cumin, paprika, salt, and pepper to the skillet. Stir and cook for an additional 2 minutes.

7. Combine the cooked quinoa, onion mixture, dried cranberries or raisins, and chopped nuts in a bowl. Adjust the seasoning if needed.

8. Once the acorn squash is roasted, stuff each half with the quinoa mixture.

9. Garnish with fresh parsley or cilantro.

For Roasted Brussels Sprouts:

1. Toss the halved Brussels sprouts with olive oil, salt, and pepper.

2. Spread them on a baking sheet and roast in the same oven as the acorn squash for the last 20 minutes or until they are crispy and golden brown.

3. Serve the quinoa-stuffed acorn squash on a plate alongside the roasted Brussels sprouts.

Spaghetti Squash with Turkey Bolognese

Ingredients:

For Spaghetti Squash:

- 1 large spaghetti squash
- Olive oil
- Salt and pepper

For Turkey Bolognese:

- 1 lb ground turkey
- 1 tablespoon olive oil
- 1 onion, finely chopped
- 2 carrots, peeled and finely chopped
- 2 celery stalks, finely chopped
- 3 cloves garlic, minced
- 1 can (28 oz) crushed tomatoes
- 1/2 cup red wine (optional)
- 2 teaspoons dried oregano
- 2 teaspoons dried basil
- 1 teaspoon dried thyme
- Salt and pepper to taste
- Grated Parmesan cheese for garnish (optional)
- Fresh basil or parsley for garnish (optional)

Instructions:

For Spaghetti Squash:

1. Preheat the oven to 375°F (190°C).

2. Cut the spaghetti squash in half lengthwise and scoop out the seeds.

3. Brush the cut sides of the squash with olive oil and season with salt and pepper.

4. Place the squash halves, cut side down, on a baking sheet.

5. Roast in the preheated oven for 40-50 minutes or until the squash is tender and can be easily shredded with a fork.

6. Once cooked, use a fork to scrape the flesh of the squash into "spaghetti" strands.

For Turkey Bolognese:

1. In a large skillet, heat olive oil over medium heat.

2. Add chopped onion, carrots, celery, and garlic. Sauté until the vegetables are softened.

3. Add ground turkey to the skillet, breaking it apart with a spatula. Cook until the turkey is browned.

4. Pour in the crushed tomatoes and red wine (if using). Stir to combine.

5. Add dried oregano, dried basil, dried thyme, salt, and pepper. Stir well.

6. Simmer the Bolognese sauce over low heat for about 20-30 minutes to allow the flavors to meld. Stir occasionally.

7. Adjust the seasoning if needed.

Assembly:

1. Serve the shredded spaghetti squash on plates or in bowls.

2. Top the spaghetti squash with a generous serving of turkey Bolognese.

3. Garnish with grated Parmesan cheese, fresh basil, or parsley if desired.

4. Serve hot and enjoy your healthy and satisfying spaghetti squash with turkey Bolognese!

Baked salmon with quinoa and steamed broccoli

Ingredients:

For Baked Salmon:

- 4 salmon filets
- 2 tablespoons olive oil
- 2 cloves garlic, minced

- 1 teaspoon lemon zest

- 2 tablespoons lemon juice

- 1 teaspoon dried oregano

- Salt and pepper to taste

- Lemon slices for garnish (optional)

- Fresh parsley for garnish (optional)

For Quinoa:

- 1 cup quinoa, rinsed

- 2 cups vegetable broth or water

- Salt to taste

For Steamed Broccoli:

- 2 cups broccoli florets

Instructions:

For Baked Salmon:

1. Preheat the oven to 375°F (190°C).

2. Place salmon filets on a baking sheet lined with parchment paper.

3. In a small bowl, whisk together olive oil, minced garlic, lemon zest, lemon juice, dried oregano, salt, and pepper.

4. Brush the salmon filets with the prepared marinade.

5. Bake in the preheated oven for 15-20 minutes or until the salmon flakes easily with a fork.

6. Optional: Garnish with lemon slices and fresh parsley before serving.

For Quinoa:

1. In a saucepan, combine quinoa and vegetable broth or water.

2. Bring to a boil, then reduce the heat to low, cover, and simmer for 15-20 minutes or until the quinoa is cooked and liquid is absorbed.

3. Fluff the quinoa with a fork and season with salt to taste.

For Steamed Broccoli:

1. Steam broccoli florets until tender-crisp, about 4-5 minutes.

2. You can steam broccoli on the stovetop or use a microwave-safe dish with a bit of water and microwave for 3-4 minutes.

Assembly:

1. Divide the cooked quinoa among serving plates.

2. Place a portion of baked salmon on top of the quinoa.

3. Arrange steamed broccoli alongside the quinoa and salmon.

4. Serve hot, garnished with additional lemon slices and fresh parsley if desired.

Turkey meatballs with whole grain pasta and roasted asparagus

Ingredients:

For Turkey Meatballs:

- 1 lb ground turkey
- 1/2 cup breadcrumbs (whole wheat if available)
- 1/4 cup grated Parmesan cheese
- 1/4 cup chopped fresh parsley
- 1 egg
- 2 cloves garlic, minced
- 1 teaspoon dried oregano
- Salt and pepper to taste
- Olive oil for baking

For Whole Grain Pasta:

- 8 oz whole grain pasta (spaghetti, penne, or your choice)
- Salt for boiling

For Roasted Asparagus:

- 1 bunch asparagus, trimmed

- 2 tablespoons olive oil
- Salt and pepper to taste

For Tomato Sauce (Optional):

- 1 can (14 oz) crushed tomatoes
- 2 cloves garlic, minced
- 1 teaspoon dried basil
- 1 teaspoon dried oregano
- Salt and pepper to taste

Instructions:

For Turkey Meatballs:

1. Preheat the oven to 375°F (190°C).
2. In a large bowl, combine ground turkey, breadcrumbs, Parmesan cheese, chopped parsley, egg, minced garlic, dried oregano, salt, and pepper. Mix until well combined.
3. Shape the mixture into meatballs, about 1 to 1.5 inches in diameter.
4. Place the meatballs on a baking sheet lined with parchment paper.
5. Bake in the preheated oven for 20-25 minutes or until the meatballs are cooked through and browned on the outside.

For Whole Grain Pasta:

1. Cook the whole grain pasta according to the package instructions in a pot of salted boiling water.
2. Drain the pasta and set aside.

For Roasted Asparagus:

1. Preheat the oven to 400°F (200°C).
2. Place trimmed asparagus on a baking sheet.
3. Drizzle with olive oil, sprinkle with salt and pepper, and toss to coat.
4. Roast in the preheated oven for 12-15 minutes or until the asparagus is tender yet still crisp.

For Tomato Sauce (Optional):

1. In a saucepan, combine crushed tomatoes, minced garlic, dried basil, dried oregano, salt, and pepper.
2. Simmer the sauce over low heat for 10-15 minutes.

Assembly:

1. In a large serving dish, arrange the cooked whole grain pasta.
2. Top the pasta with the roasted turkey meatballs.

3. Place the roasted asparagus alongside the pasta and meatballs.

4. If using, spoon tomato sauce over the meatballs.

5. Serve hot and enjoy your delicious and nutritious meal!

Grilled shrimp with quinoa and sautéed spinach

Ingredients:

For Grilled Shrimp:

- 1 lb large shrimp, peeled and deveined
- 2 tablespoons olive oil
- 2 cloves garlic, minced
- 1 teaspoon smoked paprika
- 1 teaspoon lemon zest
- Salt and pepper to taste
- Lemon wedges for serving

For Quinoa:

- 1 cup quinoa, rinsed
- 2 cups vegetable broth or water
- Salt to taste

For Sautéed Spinach:

- 8 oz fresh spinach leaves, washed and stems removed
- 2 tablespoons olive oil
- 2 cloves garlic, minced
- Salt and pepper to taste
- Crushed red pepper flakes (optional)

Instructions:

For Grilled Shrimp:

1. In a bowl, combine shrimp, olive oil, minced garlic, smoked paprika, lemon zest, salt, and pepper. Toss until the shrimp are well coated.
2. Preheat the grill or grill pan over medium-high heat.
3. Thread the shrimp onto skewers if using.
4. Grill the shrimp for 2-3 minutes per side or until they are opaque and cooked through.
5. Remove the shrimp from the grill and set aside.

For Quinoa:

1. In a saucepan, combine quinoa and vegetable broth or water.

2. Bring to a boil, then reduce the heat to low, cover, and simmer for 15-20 minutes or until the quinoa is cooked and the liquid is absorbed.

3. Fluff the quinoa with a fork and season with salt to taste.

For Sautéed Spinach:

1. In a large skillet, heat olive oil over medium heat.

2. Add minced garlic and sauté for about 1 minute or until fragrant.

3. Add fresh spinach to the skillet. Cook, stirring frequently, until the spinach wilts.

4. Season with salt, pepper, and optional crushed red pepper flakes.

Assembly:

1. Arrange a serving of quinoa on each plate.

2. Top the quinoa with grilled shrimp.

3. Spoon sautéed spinach alongside the shrimp.

4. Serve hot with lemon wedges on the side.

5. Enjoy your delicious and healthy meal!

Baked tilapia with wild rice and steamed asparagus

Ingredients:

For Baked Tilapia:

- 4 tilapia filets
- 2 tablespoons olive oil
- 2 cloves garlic, minced
- 1 teaspoon lemon zest
- 2 tablespoons lemon juice
- 1 teaspoon dried thyme
- Salt and pepper to taste
- Lemon slices for garnish (optional)
- Fresh parsley for garnish (optional)

For Wild Rice:

- 1 cup wild rice
- 3 cups vegetable broth or water
- Salt to taste

For Steamed Asparagus:

- 1 bunch asparagus, trimmed
- 2 tablespoons olive oil
- Salt and pepper to taste

Instructions:

For Baked Tilapia:

1. Preheat the oven to 400°F (200°C).

2. Place tilapia filets in a baking dish.

3. In a small bowl, mix together olive oil, minced garlic, lemon zest, lemon juice, dried thyme, salt, and pepper.

4. Brush the tilapia filets with the prepared mixture.

5. Bake in the preheated oven for 12-15 minutes or until the tilapia is cooked through and flakes easily.

6. Optional: Garnish with lemon slices and fresh parsley before serving.

For Wild Rice:

1. Rinse the wild rice under cold water.

2. In a saucepan, combine wild rice and vegetable broth or water.

3. Bring to a boil, then reduce the heat to low, cover, and simmer for 45-55 minutes or until the rice is cooked and liquid is absorbed.

4. Fluff the wild rice with a fork and season with salt to taste.

For Steamed Asparagus:

1. Bring a pot of water to a boil.

2. Place trimmed asparagus in a steamer basket.

3. Steam the asparagus for 3-5 minutes or until they are tender-crisp.

4. Drizzle with olive oil, and season with salt and pepper.

Assembly:

1. Arrange a serving of wild rice on each plate.

2. Place a baked tilapia filet on top of the wild rice.

3. Serve steamed asparagus alongside the tilapia and rice.

4. Enjoy your wholesome and flavorful meal!

Grilled vegetable and tofu skewers with couscous

Ingredients:

For Grilled Vegetable and Tofu Skewers:

- 1 block firm tofu, pressed and cubed

- 2 zucchinis, sliced

- 1 red bell pepper, cut into chunks

- 1 yellow bell pepper, cut into chunks

- 1 red onion, cut into chunks
- Cherry tomatoes
- 2 tablespoons olive oil
- 2 cloves garlic, minced
- 1 teaspoon dried oregano
- 1 teaspoon dried thyme
- Salt and pepper to taste
- Wooden skewers, soaked in water for 30 minutes

For Couscous:

- 1 cup couscous
- 1 cup vegetable broth or water
- 2 tablespoons olive oil
- 1/4 cup fresh parsley, chopped
- Salt and pepper to taste

For Lemon-Tahini Sauce (Optional):

- 1/4 cup tahini
- 2 tablespoons lemon juice
- 1 tablespoon olive oil
- 1 clove garlic, minced
- Salt and pepper to taste
- Water, as needed to thin

Instructions:

For Grilled Vegetable and Tofu Skewers:

1. In a bowl, combine cubed tofu, sliced zucchini, bell pepper chunks, red onion chunks, cherry tomatoes, olive oil, minced garlic, dried oregano, dried thyme, salt, and pepper. Toss until well coated.

2. Thread the marinated tofu and vegetables onto the soaked wooden skewers.

3. Preheat the grill or grill pan over medium-high heat.

4. Grill the skewers for 10-15 minutes, turning occasionally, until the vegetables are charred and the tofu is golden brown.

For Couscous:

1. In a saucepan, bring vegetable broth or water to a boil.

2. Stir in couscous, cover, and remove from heat. Let it sit for 5 minutes.

3. Fluff the couscous with a fork. Stir in olive oil, chopped fresh parsley, salt, and pepper.

For Lemon-Tahini Sauce (Optional):

1. In a small bowl, whisk together tahini, lemon juice, olive oil, minced garlic, salt, and pepper.

2. Add water gradually and whisk until you achieve your desired consistency.

Assembly:

1. Serve the grilled vegetable and tofu skewers on a bed of couscous.
2. Drizzle with optional lemon-tahini sauce.
3. Garnish with additional fresh parsley.
4. Enjoy your delicious and plant-based meal!

Baked cod with lemon–dill sauce, sweet potato, and green beans

Baked Cod Ingredients:

- 4 cod filets
- 2 tablespoons olive oil
- Salt and pepper to taste
- 1 teaspoon garlic powder
- 1 teaspoon dried oregano
- 1 lemon (sliced for garnish)

Lemon-Dill Sauce Ingredients:

- 1/2 cup plain Greek yogurt
- 2 tablespoons fresh dill (chopped)
- 1 tablespoon lemon juice

- Salt and pepper to taste

Sweet Potatoes and Green Beans Ingredients:

- 2 large sweet potatoes (peeled and cut into cubes)
- 1 pound fresh green beans (trimmed)
- 2 tablespoons olive oil
- Salt and pepper to taste
- 1 teaspoon paprika

Instructions:

Baked Cod:

1. Preheat your oven to 400°F (200°C).
2. Pat the cod filets dry with paper towels and place them on a baking sheet lined with parchment paper.
3. Drizzle the cod filets with olive oil, then season with salt, pepper, garlic powder, and dried oregano.
4. Place lemon slices on top of the cod filets for added flavor.
5. Bake in the preheated oven for 15-20 minutes or until the cod is opaque and flakes easily with a fork.

Lemon-Dill Sauce:

1. In a small bowl, mix together the Greek yogurt, chopped dill, lemon juice, salt, and pepper.
2. Adjust the seasoning to taste and set aside.

Sweet Potatoes and Green Beans:

1. In a large bowl, toss the sweet potato cubes and green beans with olive oil, salt, pepper, and paprika until well coated.
2. Spread the sweet potatoes and green beans on a baking sheet in a single layer.
3. Roast in the oven for about 25-30 minutes or until the sweet potatoes are tender and the green beans are crisp-tender.

Serving:

1. Plate the baked cod filets, arranging them with a side of roasted sweet potatoes and green beans.
2. Drizzle the lemon-dill sauce over the cod filets.
3. Garnish with additional fresh dill and lemon slices if desired.
4. Serve immediately and enjoy your delicious and nutritious meal!

Grilled salmon with quinoa pilaf and steamed broccoli

Grilled Salmon Ingredients:

- 4 salmon filets
- 2 tablespoons olive oil
- 2 cloves garlic (minced)
- 1 teaspoon lemon zest
- 2 tablespoons fresh lemon juice
- Salt and pepper to taste
- 1 teaspoon dried dill (optional)

Quinoa Pilaf Ingredients:

- 1 cup quinoa (rinsed)
- 2 cups vegetable or chicken broth
- 1 tablespoon olive oil
- 1 small onion (finely chopped)
- 2 cloves garlic (minced)
- 1/2 cup carrots (diced)
- 1/2 cup peas (fresh or frozen)
- Salt and pepper to taste
- 1/4 cup fresh parsley (chopped, for garnish)

Steamed Broccoli Ingredients:

- 4 cups broccoli florets

- Salt and pepper to taste
- Lemon wedges for serving

Instructions:

Grilled Salmon:

1. In a bowl, mix together olive oil, minced garlic, lemon zest, lemon juice, salt, pepper, and dried dill (if using).
2. Place the salmon filets in a shallow dish and coat them with the marinade. Let them marinate for at least 15-30 minutes.
3. Preheat the grill to medium-high heat.
4. Grill the salmon filets for about 4-5 minutes per side or until the fish flakes easily with a fork.

Quinoa Pilaf:

1. In a saucepan, heat olive oil over medium heat. Add chopped onions and garlic, sautéing until softened.
2. Add quinoa to the saucepan and cook for 2-3 minutes, stirring frequently.
3. Pour in the broth, bring to a boil, then reduce the heat to low, cover, and simmer for 15-20 minutes or until the quinoa is cooked and the liquid is absorbed.

4. In the last 5 minutes of cooking, add diced carrots and peas. Stir gently to combine.

5. Season with salt and pepper to taste. Garnish with chopped fresh parsley.

Steamed Broccoli:

1. Steam broccoli florets until they are bright green and tender-crisp. This typically takes about 5-7 minutes.

2. Season the steamed broccoli with salt and pepper.

Serving:

1. Arrange a portion of quinoa pilaf on each plate.

2. Place a grilled salmon filet on top of the quinoa.

3. Serve steamed broccoli on the side.

4. Garnish with additional lemon wedges and fresh parsley.

5. Enjoy your nutritious and flavorful grilled salmon with quinoa pilaf and steamed broccoli!

Turkey chili with black beans, tomatoes, and a side of whole grain rice

Turkey Chili Ingredients:

- 1 pound ground turkey
- 1 tablespoon olive oil
- 1 large onion (diced)
- 3 cloves garlic (minced)
- 1 red bell pepper (diced)
- 1 can (15 oz) black beans (drained and rinsed)
- 1 can (14 oz) diced tomatoes (with juices)
- 1 can (8 oz) tomato sauce
- 1 cup low-sodium chicken broth
- 2 tablespoons chili powder
- 1 tablespoon cumin
- 1 teaspoon paprika
- 1/2 teaspoon cayenne pepper (optional, for heat)
- Salt and pepper to taste
- Fresh cilantro or green onions for garnish (optional)

Whole Grain Rice Ingredients:

- 2 cups whole grain rice

- 4 cups water or chicken broth
- Salt to taste

Instructions:

Turkey Chili:

1. In a large pot, heat olive oil over medium heat. Add diced onions and cook until softened.

2. Add minced garlic and diced red bell pepper. Sauté for an additional 2-3 minutes.

3. Add ground turkey to the pot, breaking it up with a spoon. Cook until the turkey is browned and cooked through.

4. Stir in chili powder, cumin, paprika, and cayenne pepper (if using). Cook for 1-2 minutes to allow the spices to bloom.

5. Add black beans, diced tomatoes (with juices), tomato sauce, and chicken broth to the pot. Stir well to combine.

6. Season with salt and pepper to taste. Bring the chili to a simmer, then reduce the heat to low, cover, and let it simmer for at least 20-30 minutes to allow the flavors to meld.

7. While the chili is simmering, prepare the whole grain rice.

Whole Grain Rice:

1. Rinse the whole grain rice under cold water until the water runs clear.

2. In a saucepan, combine the rice, water or chicken broth, and a pinch of salt. Bring to a boil.

3. Reduce the heat to low, cover, and simmer for about 45-50 minutes or until the rice is tender and the liquid is absorbed.

4. Fluff the rice with a fork before serving.

Serving:

1. Spoon a generous portion of the turkey chili into bowls.

2. Serve the chili over a bed of whole grain rice.

3. Garnish with fresh cilantro or green onions if desired.

4. Enjoy your hearty and wholesome turkey chili with black beans, tomatoes, and whole grain rice!

Stir-fried tofu with broccoli, bell peppers, and brown rice

Tofu Stir-Fry Ingredients:

- 1 block (14 oz) extra-firm tofu, pressed and cubed
- 3 tablespoons soy sauce
- 2 tablespoons hoisin sauce
- 1 tablespoon rice vinegar
- 1 tablespoon sesame oil
- 1 tablespoon cornstarch
- 2 tablespoons vegetable oil (for stir-frying)
- 3 cups broccoli florets
- 1 red bell pepper, thinly sliced
- 1 yellow bell pepper, thinly sliced
- 3 cloves garlic, minced
- 1 tablespoon fresh ginger, grated
- 2 green onions, sliced (for garnish)
- Sesame seeds (for garnish, optional)

Brown Rice:

- 2 cups brown rice
- 4 cups water
- 1/2 teaspoon salt

Instructions:

Brown Rice:

1. Rinse the brown rice under cold water until the water runs clear.
2. In a saucepan, combine the rice, water, and salt. Bring to a boil.
3. Reduce the heat to low, cover, and simmer for about 45-50 minutes or until the rice is tender and the liquid is absorbed.
4. Fluff the rice with a fork before serving.

Tofu Stir-Fry:

1. In a bowl, whisk together soy sauce, hoisin sauce, rice vinegar, sesame oil, and cornstarch to create the marinade.
2. Toss the cubed tofu in the marinade, ensuring each piece is well coated. Let it marinate for at least 15-30 minutes.
3. Heat 2 tablespoons of vegetable oil in a large wok or skillet over medium-high heat.
4. Add marinated tofu cubes and cook until they are golden brown on all sides. Remove tofu from the pan and set aside.

5. In the same pan, add another tablespoon of oil if needed. Add minced garlic and grated ginger, sauté for about 1 minute until fragrant.

6. Add broccoli florets and bell peppers to the pan. Stir-fry for 3-5 minutes until the vegetables are tender-crisp.

7. Return the cooked tofu to the pan and toss everything together to combine.

8. Cook for an additional 2-3 minutes until the tofu is heated through.

Serving:

1. Serve the stir-fried tofu, broccoli, and bell peppers over a bed of brown rice.

2. Garnish with sliced green onions and sesame seeds if desired.

3. Enjoy this delicious and nutritious stir-fried tofu with broccoli, bell peppers, and brown rice!

Baked chicken breast with quinoa pilaf and steamed broccoli

Baked Chicken Breast Ingredients:

- 4 boneless, skinless chicken breasts
- 2 tablespoons olive oil

- 1 teaspoon garlic powder
- 1 teaspoon paprika
- 1 teaspoon dried thyme
- Salt and pepper to taste
- Lemon wedges for serving

Quinoa Pilaf Ingredients:

- 1 cup quinoa, rinsed
- 2 cups chicken broth
- 1 tablespoon olive oil
- 1 small onion, finely chopped
- 2 cloves garlic, minced
- 1/2 cup carrots, diced
- 1/2 cup peas (fresh or frozen)
- Salt and pepper to taste
- 2 tablespoons chopped fresh parsley (for garnish)

Steamed Broccoli:

- 4 cups broccoli florets
- Salt and pepper to taste

Instructions:

Baked Chicken Breast:

1. Preheat the oven to 400°F (200°C).

2. Place the chicken breasts on a baking sheet lined with parchment paper.

3. In a small bowl, mix together olive oil, garlic powder, paprika, dried thyme, salt, and pepper.

4. Brush the chicken breasts with the olive oil mixture, ensuring they are well-coated.

5. Bake in the preheated oven for about 20-25 minutes or until the internal temperature reaches 165°F (74°C) and the chicken is cooked through.

6. Once baked, let the chicken rest for a few minutes before slicing.

Quinoa Pilaf:

1. In a saucepan, heat olive oil over medium heat. Add chopped onions and cook until softened.

2. Add minced garlic and cook for an additional 1-2 minutes.

3. Add quinoa to the saucepan and cook for 2-3 minutes, stirring frequently.

4. Pour in the chicken broth, bring to a boil, then reduce the heat to low, cover, and simmer for 15-20 minutes or until the quinoa is cooked and the liquid is absorbed.

5. In the last 5 minutes of cooking, add diced carrots and peas. Stir gently to combine.

6. Season with salt and pepper to taste. Garnish with chopped fresh parsley.

Steamed Broccoli:

1. Steam broccoli florets until they are bright green and tender-crisp. This typically takes about 5-7 minutes.

2. Season the steamed broccoli with salt and pepper.

Serving:

1. Place a portion of quinoa pilaf on each plate.

2. Top with slices of baked chicken breast.

3. Serve steamed broccoli on the side.

4. Garnish with lemon wedges.

5. Enjoy your balanced and wholesome meal of baked chicken breast with quinoa pilaf and steamed broccoli!

Grilled cod with quinoa and roasted Brussels sprouts

Grilled Cod Ingredients:

- 4 cod filets
- 2 tablespoons olive oil
- 1 teaspoon lemon zest

- 2 tablespoons fresh lemon juice
- 2 cloves garlic, minced
- 1 teaspoon dried oregano
- Salt and pepper to taste
- Lemon wedges for serving

Quinoa Ingredients:

1. 1 cup quinoa, rinsed
2. 2 cups vegetable or chicken broth
3. 1 tablespoon olive oil
4. Salt to taste
5. 2 tablespoons chopped fresh parsley (for garnish)

Roasted Brussels Sprouts Ingredients:

- 1 pound Brussels sprouts, trimmed and halved
- 2 tablespoons olive oil
- Salt and pepper to taste
- 1 teaspoon garlic powder
- 1/4 cup grated Parmesan cheese (optional, for garnish)

Instructions:

Grilled Cod:

1. Preheat the grill to medium-high heat.

2. In a bowl, whisk together olive oil, lemon zest, lemon juice, minced garlic, dried oregano, salt, and pepper to create a marinade.

3. Pat the cod filets dry with paper towels and coat them with the marinade. Let them marinate for about 15-30 minutes.

4. Grill the cod filets for about 4-5 minutes per side or until the fish is opaque and easily flakes with a fork.

5. Remove the cod from the grill and set aside.

Quinoa:

1. In a saucepan, heat olive oil over medium heat. Add quinoa and toast for 2-3 minutes, stirring frequently.

2. Pour in the broth, bring to a boil, then reduce the heat to low, cover, and simmer for 15-20 minutes or until the quinoa is cooked and the liquid is absorbed.

3. Fluff the quinoa with a fork and season with salt to taste.

4. Garnish with chopped fresh parsley.

Roasted Brussels Sprouts:

1. Preheat the oven to 400°F (200°C).

2. Toss halved Brussels sprouts with olive oil, salt, pepper, and garlic powder on a baking sheet.

3. Roast in the preheated oven for 20-25 minutes or until the Brussels sprouts are golden brown and crispy on the edges.

4. Optional: Sprinkle grated Parmesan cheese over the roasted Brussels sprouts during the last 5 minutes of cooking.

Serving:

1. Place a portion of quinoa on each plate.

2. Top with a grilled cod filet.

3. Serve roasted Brussels sprouts on the side.

4. Garnish with lemon wedges.

5. Enjoy your flavorful and nutritious meal of grilled cod with quinoa and roasted Brussels sprouts!

Grilled chicken with wild rice and steamed asparagus

Grilled Chicken Ingredients:

- 4 boneless, skinless chicken breasts
- 2 tablespoons olive oil
- 2 teaspoons dried thyme

- 1 teaspoon paprika
- 1 teaspoon garlic powder
- Salt and pepper to taste
- Lemon wedges for serving

Wild Rice Ingredients:

- 1 cup wild rice
- 3 cups chicken broth
- 1 tablespoon unsalted butter
- Salt and pepper to taste
- Chopped fresh parsley (for garnish)

Steamed Asparagus Ingredients:

- 1 pound fresh asparagus, trimmed
- 1 tablespoon olive oil
- Salt and pepper to taste
- Lemon zest (optional, for garnish)

Instructions:

Grilled Chicken:

1. Preheat the grill to medium-high heat.
2. In a bowl, mix together olive oil, dried thyme, paprika, garlic powder, salt, and pepper to create a marinade.
3. Brush the chicken breasts with the marinade, ensuring they are well-coated.

4. Grill the chicken breasts for approximately 6-8 minutes per side or until they reach an internal temperature of 165°F (74°C) and have nice grill marks.

5. Remove the chicken from the grill and let it rest for a few minutes before slicing.

Wild Rice:

1. Rinse the wild rice under cold water.

2. In a saucepan, combine the wild rice and chicken broth. Bring to a boil.

3. Reduce the heat to low, cover, and simmer for about 40-45 minutes or until the rice is tender and the liquid is absorbed.

4. Stir in unsalted butter and season with salt and pepper to taste.

5. Garnish with chopped fresh parsley.

Steamed Asparagus:

1. Steam the trimmed asparagus for 3-5 minutes or until they are bright green and tender-crisp.

2. Drizzle with olive oil and season with salt and pepper.

3. Optional: Garnish with lemon zest for an extra burst of flavor.

Serving:

1. Place a portion of wild rice on each plate.

2. Top with sliced grilled chicken breasts.

3. Arrange steamed asparagus on the side.

4. Garnish with lemon wedges.

5. Enjoy your delicious and wholesome meal of grilled chicken with wild rice and steamed asparagus!

Beef and vegetable kebabs with sweet potato wedges

Beef and Vegetable Kebabs Ingredients:

- 1.5 pounds beef sirloin or your preferred beef cut, cut into cubes
- 1 red bell pepper, cut into chunks
- 1 yellow bell pepper, cut into chunks
- 1 red onion, cut into chunks
- Cherry tomatoes
- 2 tablespoons olive oil
- 2 cloves garlic, minced
- 1 teaspoon dried oregano
- 1 teaspoon paprika

- Salt and pepper to taste
- Metal or bamboo skewers (if using bamboo, soak them in water for 30 minutes)

Sweet Potato Wedges Ingredients:

- 2 large sweet potatoes, peeled and cut into wedges
- 2 tablespoons olive oil
- 1 teaspoon smoked paprika
- 1 teaspoon garlic powder
- Salt and pepper to taste

Instructions:

Beef and Vegetable Kebabs:

1. In a bowl, combine olive oil, minced garlic, dried oregano, paprika, salt, and pepper to create a marinade.
2. Place the beef cubes in the marinade and let them marinate for at least 30 minutes, or longer for more flavor.
3. Preheat the grill to medium-high heat.
4. Thread the marinated beef cubes, bell peppers, red onion, and cherry tomatoes onto skewers, alternating the ingredients.

5. Grill the kebabs for about 10-12 minutes, turning occasionally, until the beef is cooked to your liking and the vegetables are charred and tender.

Sweet Potato Wedges:

1. Preheat the oven to 425°F (220°C).

2. In a large bowl, toss the sweet potato wedges with olive oil, smoked paprika, garlic powder, salt, and pepper until evenly coated.

3. Arrange the sweet potato wedges on a baking sheet in a single layer.

4. Bake in the preheated oven for 25-30 minutes or until the sweet potatoes are golden brown and tender, flipping them halfway through.

Serving:

1. Serve the beef and vegetable kebabs on a platter.

2. Place the sweet potato wedges alongside the kebabs.

3. Garnish with additional fresh herbs if desired.

4. Enjoy your delicious and satisfying meal of beef and vegetable kebabs with sweet potato wedges!

Baked chicken thighs with sweet potato mash and green beans

Baked Chicken Thighs Ingredients:

- 8 bone-in, skin-on chicken thighs
- 2 tablespoons olive oil
- 1 teaspoon garlic powder
- 1 teaspoon smoked paprika
- 1 teaspoon dried thyme
- Salt and pepper to taste
- Lemon wedges for serving

Sweet Potato Mash Ingredients:

- 4 large sweet potatoes, peeled and cut into chunks
- 3 tablespoons unsalted butter
- 1/4 cup milk or cream
- Salt and pepper to taste
- Chopped fresh chives or parsley for garnish

Green Beans Ingredients:

- 1 pound fresh green beans, trimmed
- 2 tablespoons olive oil
- 2 cloves garlic, minced
- Salt and pepper to taste

- Lemon zest (optional, for garnish)

Instructions:

Baked Chicken Thighs:

1. Preheat the oven to 425°F (220°C).
2. In a small bowl, mix together olive oil, garlic powder, smoked paprika, dried thyme, salt, and pepper.
3. Pat the chicken thighs dry with paper towels and place them on a baking sheet.
4. Brush the chicken thighs with the spice mixture, ensuring they are well-coated.
5. Bake in the preheated oven for about 35-40 minutes or until the chicken reaches an internal temperature of 165°F (74°C) and the skin is crispy.
6. Serve with lemon wedges on the side.

Sweet Potato Mash:

1. In a large pot, bring water to a boil. Add sweet potato chunks and cook until tender, about 15-20 minutes.
2. Drain the sweet potatoes and return them to the pot.
3. Mash the sweet potatoes with butter, milk or cream until smooth and creamy.

4. Season with salt and pepper to taste.

5. Garnish with chopped fresh chives or parsley.

Green Beans:

1. Steam or blanch the green beans until they are bright green and tender-crisp, about 3-5 minutes.

2. In a skillet, heat olive oil over medium heat. Add minced garlic and sauté for about 1 minute.

3. Add the steamed green beans to the skillet and toss to coat in the garlic-infused oil.

4. Season with salt and pepper to taste.

5. Optional: Garnish with lemon zest for an extra burst of flavor.

Serving:

1. Place a generous scoop of sweet potato mash on each plate.

2. Arrange baked chicken thighs on top.

3. Serve the green beans alongside.

4. Garnish with additional herbs and lemon zest if desired.

5. Enjoy your comforting and flavorful meal of baked chicken thighs with sweet potato mash and green beans!

"My commitment to a healthy lifestyle is strengthening my liver."

"I am patient with my body as it heals and restores balance."

CHAPTER 7: FISH AND SEAFOOD RECIPES

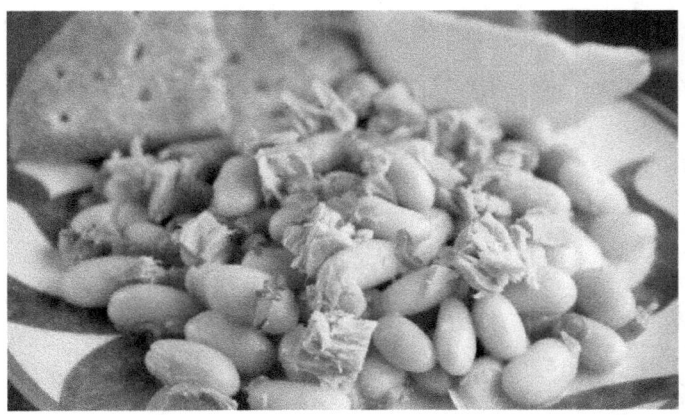

Baked Cod with Herbs

Ingredients:

- 4 cod filets (about 6 ounces each)
- 2 tablespoons olive oil
- 2 tablespoons fresh lemon juice
- 2 cloves garlic, minced
- 1 teaspoon dried oregano
- 1 teaspoon dried thyme
- 1 teaspoon dried rosemary
- Salt and black pepper, to taste

- Lemon wedges for serving
- Fresh parsley, chopped, for garnish

Instructions:

1. Preheat your oven to 400°F (200°C). Line a baking sheet with parchment paper or lightly grease it.

2. In a small bowl, whisk together the olive oil, lemon juice, minced garlic, oregano, thyme, rosemary, salt, and black pepper.

3. Place the cod filets on the prepared baking sheet.

4. Brush the cod filets with the herb mixture, ensuring they are well coated on both sides.

5. Bake in the preheated oven for about 15-20 minutes or until the cod is cooked through and easily flakes with a fork.

6. If desired, you can broil the cod for an additional 2-3 minutes to achieve a golden crust on top.

7. Remove the baked cod from the oven, garnish with fresh parsley, and serve with lemon wedges on the side.

8. Enjoy your Baked Cod with Herbs as a flavorful and light main dish.

Garlic and Herb Shrimp Skewers

Ingredients:

- 1 pound large shrimp, peeled and deveined
- 3 cloves garlic, minced
- 2 tablespoons fresh parsley, chopped
- 1 tablespoon fresh cilantro, chopped
- 2 tablespoons olive oil
- 1 tablespoon lemon juice
- 1 teaspoon paprika
- 1/2 teaspoon dried oregano
- 1/2 teaspoon dried thyme
- Salt and black pepper, to taste
- Lemon wedges for serving

Instructions:

1. In a bowl, mix together minced garlic, chopped parsley, chopped cilantro, olive oil, lemon juice, paprika, dried oregano, dried thyme, salt, and black pepper.

2. Add the peeled and deveined shrimp to the marinade, ensuring they are well coated. Allow the shrimp to marinate for at least 15-20 minutes in the refrigerator.

3. Preheat your grill or grill pan over medium-high heat.

4. Thread the marinated shrimp onto skewers.

5. Grill the shrimp skewers for about 2-3 minutes per side or until they are opaque and cooked through. Be careful not to overcook, as shrimp cook quickly.

6. Remove the shrimp skewers from the grill.

7. Serve the Garlic and Herb Shrimp Skewers with lemon wedges on the side.

8. Enjoy your delicious and aromatic shrimp skewers as a main dish or as part of a seafood feast.

Tuna and White Bean Salad

Ingredients:

- 1 can (15 ounces) white beans (cannellini or Great Northern), drained and rinsed
- 1 can (5 ounces) tuna, drained
- 1/2 red onion, finely chopped
- 1/2 cup cherry tomatoes, halved
- 1/4 cup Kalamata olives, pitted and sliced
- 2 tablespoons fresh parsley, chopped

- 2 tablespoons extra-virgin olive oil
- 1 tablespoon red wine vinegar
- Salt and black pepper, to taste
- Lemon wedges for serving (optional)

Instructions:

1. In a large bowl, combine the white beans, tuna, chopped red onion, cherry tomatoes, Kalamata olives, and chopped parsley.

2. In a small bowl, whisk together the extra-virgin olive oil and red wine vinegar. Season with salt and black pepper to taste.

3. Pour the dressing over the bean and tuna mixture. Gently toss until all ingredients are well coated.

4. Taste and adjust the seasoning if necessary.

5. Allow the salad to marinate in the refrigerator for at least 15-20 minutes to let the flavors meld.

6. Serve the Tuna and White Bean Salad on a platter or individual plates. Optionally, squeeze lemon wedges over the salad before serving.

7. Enjoy this protein-packed and flavorful salad as a light meal or a satisfying side dish.

Lemon Garlic Tilapia

Ingredients:

- 4 tilapia filets
- 2 tablespoons olive oil
- 3 cloves garlic, minced
- 1 teaspoon lemon zest
- 2 tablespoons fresh lemon juice
- 1 teaspoon dried oregano
- Salt and black pepper, to taste
- Fresh parsley, chopped, for garnish
- Lemon wedges for serving

Instructions:

1. Preheat your oven to 375°F (190°C).
2. Place the tilapia filets in a baking dish.
3. In a small bowl, whisk together the olive oil, minced garlic, lemon zest, lemon juice, dried oregano, salt, and black pepper.
4. Pour the lemon garlic mixture over the tilapia filets, ensuring they are well coated on both sides.
5. Bake in the preheated oven for about 12-15 minutes or until the tilapia is cooked through and easily flakes with a fork.

6. If you prefer a golden crust on top, you can broil the tilapia for an additional 2-3 minutes.

7. Remove the Lemon Garlic Tilapia from the oven, sprinkle with fresh chopped parsley, and serve with lemon wedges on the side.

8. Enjoy this flavorful and light dish as a main course.

Baked Halibut with Mango Salsa

Ingredients:

For the Baked Halibut:

- 4 halibut filets (about 6 ounces each)
- 2 tablespoons olive oil
- 2 tablespoons fresh lime juice
- 2 cloves garlic, minced
- 1 teaspoon ground cumin
- Salt and black pepper, to taste

For the Mango Salsa:

- 1 ripe mango, peeled, pitted, and diced
- 1/2 red onion, finely chopped
- 1 jalapeño, seeds removed and finely chopped
- 1/4 cup fresh cilantro, chopped
- 1 tablespoon fresh lime juice

- Salt and black pepper, to taste

Instructions:

1. Preheat your oven to 400°F (200°C).

2. In a small bowl, whisk together olive oil, fresh lime juice, minced garlic, ground cumin, salt, and black pepper.

3. Place the halibut filets in a baking dish. Pour the lime and cumin mixture over the filets, ensuring they are well coated. Let them marinate for about 15 minutes.

4. Bake the halibut in the preheated oven for approximately 15-20 minutes, or until the fish flakes easily with a fork.

5. While the halibut is baking, prepare the mango salsa. In a bowl, combine diced mango, chopped red onion, chopped jalapeño, chopped cilantro, fresh lime juice, salt, and black pepper. Mix well.

6. Once the halibut is done, remove it from the oven.

7. Serve the Baked Halibut on plates, topped with generous spoonfuls of Mango Salsa.

8. Garnish with additional cilantro and lime wedges if desired.

9. Enjoy this flavorful and colorful dish that combines the mildness of halibut with the sweet and tangy mango salsa.

Mediterranean Grilled Swordfish

Ingredients:

For the Swordfish Marinade:

- 4 swordfish steaks (about 6-8 ounces each)
- 1/4 cup olive oil
- 3 tablespoons fresh lemon juice
- 2 cloves garlic, minced
- 1 teaspoon dried oregano
- 1 teaspoon dried thyme
- Salt and black pepper, to taste

For the Mediterranean Salsa:

- 1 cup cherry tomatoes, halved
- 1/2 cucumber, diced
- 1/4 cup Kalamata olives, pitted and sliced
- 1/4 cup red onion, finely chopped
- 1/4 cup feta cheese, crumbled
- 2 tablespoons fresh lemon juice
- 2 tablespoons extra-virgin olive oil
- 1 tablespoon fresh parsley, chopped

- Salt and black pepper, to taste

Instructions:

1. In a bowl, whisk together the olive oil, fresh lemon juice, minced garlic, dried oregano, dried thyme, salt, and black pepper to create the marinade.

2. Place the swordfish steaks in a shallow dish and pour the marinade over them. Ensure that each steak is well coated. Marinate in the refrigerator for at least 30 minutes.

3. Preheat your grill to medium-high heat.

4. While the grill is heating, prepare the Mediterranean salsa. In a bowl, combine cherry tomatoes, diced cucumber, sliced Kalamata olives, finely chopped red onion, crumbled feta cheese, fresh lemon juice, extra-virgin olive oil, chopped parsley, salt, and black pepper. Toss gently to combine.

5. Remove the swordfish from the marinade and let any excess marinade drip off.

6. Grill the swordfish steaks for about 4-5 minutes per side or until they are cooked through and have distinct grill marks.

7. Serve the grilled swordfish steaks topped with the Mediterranean salsa.

8. Garnish with additional parsley and lemon wedges if desired.

9. Enjoy this Mediterranean Grilled Swordfish as a flavorful and healthy main course.

Cajun Shrimp and Quinoa

Ingredients:

For the Cajun Shrimp:

- 1 pound large shrimp, peeled and deveined
- 1 tablespoon Cajun seasoning
- 1 tablespoon olive oil
- 2 cloves garlic, minced
- Salt and black pepper, to taste
- Lemon wedges for serving

For the Quinoa:

- 1 cup quinoa, rinsed
- 2 cups vegetable or chicken broth
- 1 tablespoon olive oil
- 1 small onion, finely chopped
- 1 bell pepper (any color), diced
- 2 celery stalks, diced

- 2 cloves garlic, minced
- 1 teaspoon Cajun seasoning
- Salt and black pepper, to taste
- Fresh parsley, chopped, for garnish

Instructions:

1. In a bowl, toss the peeled and deveined shrimp with Cajun seasoning, olive oil, minced garlic, salt, and black pepper. Allow the shrimp to marinate for at least 15 minutes.

2. Rinse the quinoa under cold water.

3. In a medium saucepan, heat olive oil over medium heat. Add chopped onion, diced bell pepper, diced celery, and minced garlic. Sauté until the vegetables are softened.

4. Add the rinsed quinoa to the saucepan and stir for 1-2 minutes to toast the quinoa.

5. Pour in the vegetable or chicken broth, add Cajun seasoning, salt, and black pepper. Bring the mixture to a boil, then reduce the heat to low, cover, and simmer for about 15 minutes or until the quinoa is cooked and the liquid is absorbed. Fluff the quinoa with a fork.

6. While the quinoa is cooking, heat a skillet over medium-high heat. Add the marinated shrimp and cook for about 2-3 minutes per side or until they are opaque and cooked through.

7. Serve the Cajun Shrimp over a bed of Cajun Quinoa.

8. Garnish with fresh chopped parsley and serve with lemon wedges on the side.

9. Enjoy this flavorful and spicy Cajun Shrimp and Quinoa dish.

Seared Scallops with Citrus Glaze

Ingredients:

For the Seared Scallops:

- 1 pound sea scallops, side muscle removed
- Salt and black pepper, to taste
- 2 tablespoons olive oil
- 1 tablespoon unsalted butter

For the Citrus Glaze:

- 1/2 cup orange juice
- 1/4 cup lemon juice
- 2 tablespoons honey
- 1 tablespoon soy sauce

- 1 teaspoon grated fresh ginger
- 2 cloves garlic, minced
- 1 teaspoon cornstarch mixed with 1 tablespoon water (optional, for thickening)

Instructions:

1. Pat the scallops dry with paper towels. Season them with salt and black pepper on both sides.

2. In a large skillet, heat olive oil and butter over medium-high heat until hot but not smoking.

3. Add the scallops to the skillet, making sure not to overcrowd the pan. Sear for about 2-3 minutes per side or until they develop a golden-brown crust. Be careful not to overcook; scallops should be opaque in the center.

4. Remove the scallops from the skillet and set them aside.

5. In the same skillet, combine orange juice, lemon juice, honey, soy sauce, grated ginger, and minced garlic. Bring the mixture to a simmer.

6. If you prefer a thicker glaze, you can add the cornstarch-water mixture to the simmering sauce. Stir until the glaze thickens slightly.

7. Return the seared scallops to the skillet, coating them with the citrus glaze. Cook for an additional minute to heat the scallops through.

8. Serve the Seared Scallops with Citrus Glaze over rice, quinoa, or your preferred side dish.

9. Garnish with fresh herbs, such as chopped parsley or cilantro, if desired.

10. Enjoy this elegant and flavorful dish with a bright and citrusy glaze.

Teriyaki Glazed Salmon

Ingredients:

For the Teriyaki Glaze:

- 1/4 cup soy sauce
- 2 tablespoons mirin (Japanese sweet rice wine)
- 2 tablespoons sake (or white wine)
- 2 tablespoons brown sugar
- 1 tablespoon honey
- 1 teaspoon grated fresh ginger
- 2 cloves garlic, minced
- 1 tablespoon cornstarch mixed with 2 tablespoons water (optional, for thickening)

For the Salmon:

- 4 salmon filets (about 6 ounces each)
- Salt and black pepper, to taste
- 1 tablespoon vegetable oil
- Sesame seeds and sliced green onions for garnish (optional)

Instructions:

1. In a small saucepan, combine soy sauce, mirin, sake, brown sugar, honey, grated ginger, and minced garlic for the teriyaki glaze. Bring the mixture to a simmer over medium heat.

2. If you prefer a thicker glaze, you can add the cornstarch-water mixture to the simmering sauce. Stir until the glaze thickens slightly. Remove from heat.

3. Preheat your oven to 400°F (200°C).

4. Season the salmon filets with salt and black pepper.

5. Heat vegetable oil in an oven-safe skillet over medium-high heat.

6. Place the salmon filets in the skillet, skin side down, and sear for about 2-3 minutes until the skin is golden and crisp.

7. Brush the top of the salmon filets with the teriyaki glaze.

8. Transfer the skillet to the preheated oven and bake for about 8-10 minutes or until the salmon is cooked through and flakes easily with a fork.

9. During the last couple of minutes of baking, you can brush more teriyaki glaze over the salmon.

10. Once done, remove the salmon from the oven and brush with additional teriyaki glaze if desired.

11. Garnish with sesame seeds and sliced green onions, if you like.

12. Serve the Teriyaki Glazed Salmon over rice or your favorite side dish.

Baked Lemon Butter Cod

Ingredients:

- 4 cod filets (about 6 ounces each)
- Salt and black pepper, to taste
- 1/4 cup unsalted butter, melted
- 2 tablespoons fresh lemon juice
- 2 cloves garlic, minced
- 1 teaspoon lemon zest

- 1/2 teaspoon dried thyme
- 1/2 teaspoon paprika
- Fresh parsley, chopped, for garnish
- Lemon wedges for serving

Instructions:

1. Preheat your oven to 400°F (200°C). Line a baking sheet with parchment paper or lightly grease it.
2. Pat the cod filets dry with paper towels and season them with salt and black pepper on both sides.
3. In a bowl, mix together melted butter, fresh lemon juice, minced garlic, lemon zest, dried thyme, and paprika.
4. Place the cod filets on the prepared baking sheet.
5. Brush the cod filets with the lemon butter mixture, ensuring they are well coated on both sides.
6. Bake in the preheated oven for about 12-15 minutes or until the cod is cooked through and easily flakes with a fork.
7. If you prefer a golden crust on top, you can broil the cod for an additional 2-3 minutes.

8. Remove the Baked Lemon Butter Cod from the oven, sprinkle with fresh chopped parsley, and serve with lemon wedges on the side.

9. Enjoy your flavorful and light Baked Lemon Butter Cod.

Grilled Tuna Steak with Avocado Salsa

Ingredients:

For the Tuna Steak:

- 4 tuna steaks (about 6 ounces each)
- 2 tablespoons soy sauce
- 1 tablespoon olive oil
- 1 tablespoon fresh lemon juice
- 2 cloves garlic, minced
- 1 teaspoon ground cumin
- 1 teaspoon paprika
- Salt and black pepper, to taste

For the Avocado Salsa:

- 2 ripe avocados, diced
- 1 cup cherry tomatoes, halved
- 1/4 cup red onion, finely chopped
- 1/4 cup fresh cilantro, chopped
- 1 tablespoon fresh lime juice

- Salt and black pepper, to taste

Instructions:

1. In a bowl, whisk together soy sauce, olive oil, fresh lemon juice, minced garlic, ground cumin, paprika, salt, and black pepper to create the marinade for the tuna steaks.

2. Place the tuna steaks in a shallow dish and pour the marinade over them. Ensure that each steak is well coated. Marinate in the refrigerator for at least 30 minutes.

3. Preheat your grill or grill pan over medium-high heat.

4. While the grill is heating, prepare the avocado salsa. In a bowl, combine diced avocados, cherry tomatoes, chopped red onion, chopped cilantro, fresh lime juice, salt, and black pepper. Gently toss to combine.

5. Remove the tuna steaks from the marinade and let any excess marinade drip off.

6. Grill the tuna steaks for about 2-3 minutes per side for a medium-rare doneness, or adjust the cooking time to your preference.

7. Remove the grilled tuna steaks from the heat.

8. Serve the Grilled Tuna Steaks with Avocado Salsa on a platter or individual plates.

9. Spoon the avocado salsa over the tuna steaks.

10. Enjoy this flavorful and healthy dish.

Pesto Salmon Foil Packets

Ingredients:

- 4 salmon filets (about 6 ounces each)
- Salt and black pepper, to taste
- 1/2 cup pesto sauce (store-bought or homemade)
- 1 cup cherry tomatoes, halved
- 1 small zucchini, thinly sliced
- 1/2 cup red bell pepper, thinly sliced
- 4 tablespoons grated Parmesan cheese
- Fresh basil, chopped, for garnish
- Lemon wedges for serving

Instructions:

1. Preheat your oven to 400°F (200°C).

2. Place each salmon filet on a separate sheet of aluminum foil.

3. Season the salmon filets with salt and black pepper.

4. Spread a generous spoonful of pesto sauce over each salmon filet.

5. Divide the cherry tomatoes, zucchini slices, and red bell pepper slices evenly among the foil packets, arranging them around the salmon.

6. Sprinkle grated Parmesan cheese over each salmon filet.

7. Fold the edges of the foil to create sealed packets, ensuring the ingredients are well-contained.

8. Place the foil packets on a baking sheet and bake in the preheated oven for about 15-20 minutes, or until the salmon is cooked through and flakes easily.

9. Carefully open the foil packets, garnish the salmon with fresh chopped basil, and serve with lemon wedges on the side.

10. Enjoy your flavorful and hassle-free Pesto Salmon Foil Packets.

CHAPTER 8: MEAT AND POULTRY RECIPES

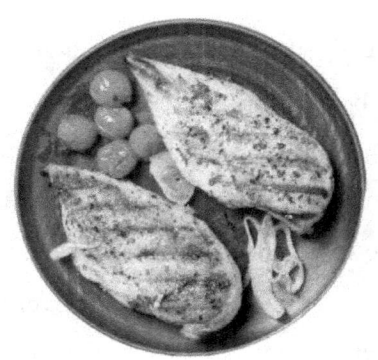

Grilled Lemon Herb Chicken Breast

Ingredients:

- 4 boneless, skinless chicken breasts
- 2 tablespoons olive oil
- Zest of 1 lemon
- Juice of 1 lemon
- 2 cloves garlic, minced
- 1 teaspoon dried thyme
- 1 teaspoon dried rosemary
- 1 teaspoon dried oregano

- Salt and black pepper, to taste
- Fresh parsley, chopped, for garnish
- Lemon wedges for serving

Instructions:

1. Preheat your grill to medium-high heat.

2. In a bowl, whisk together olive oil, lemon zest, lemon juice, minced garlic, dried thyme, dried rosemary, dried oregano, salt, and black pepper.

3. Place the chicken breasts in a shallow dish and pour the lemon herb marinade over them. Ensure that each chicken breast is well coated. Let them marinate for at least 30 minutes in the refrigerator.

4. Remove the chicken breasts from the refrigerator and let them come to room temperature for about 15 minutes.

5. Grill the chicken breasts for approximately 6-8 minutes per side or until they are fully cooked. The internal temperature should reach 165°F (74°C).

6. While grilling, you can baste the chicken with any remaining marinade for extra flavor.

7. Once done, remove the chicken from the grill and let it rest for a few minutes.

8. Sprinkle chopped fresh parsley over the grilled chicken breasts for garnish.

9. Serve the Grilled Lemon Herb Chicken Breast with lemon wedges on the side.

10. Enjoy this light and flavorful grilled chicken as a main dish, paired with your favorite sides.

Baked Turkey Meatballs with Zucchini Noodles

Ingredients:

For the Turkey Meatballs:

- 1 pound ground turkey
- 1/2 cup breadcrumbs
- 1/4 cup grated Parmesan cheese
- 1/4 cup chopped fresh parsley
- 1 egg
- 2 cloves garlic, minced
- 1 teaspoon dried oregano
- 1 teaspoon dried basil
- Salt and black pepper, to taste

For the Zucchini Noodles:

- 4 medium zucchini, spiralized into noodles

- 2 tablespoons olive oil
- Salt and black pepper, to taste

For the Tomato Sauce:

- 1 can (14 ounces) crushed tomatoes
- 2 cloves garlic, minced
- 1 teaspoon dried Italian seasoning
- Salt and black pepper, to taste

Instructions:

1. Preheat your oven to 400°F (200°C). Line a baking sheet with parchment paper.

2. In a large bowl, combine ground turkey, breadcrumbs, Parmesan cheese, chopped parsley, egg, minced garlic, dried oregano, dried basil, salt, and black pepper. Mix until well combined.

3. Shape the mixture into meatballs, about 1 to 1.5 inches in diameter, and place them on the prepared baking sheet.

4. Bake the turkey meatballs in the preheated oven for about 20-25 minutes or until they are cooked through and golden brown.

5. While the meatballs are baking, prepare the zucchini noodles. In a large skillet, heat olive oil over medium heat. Add the spiralized zucchini noodles and sauté for 3-5 minutes until they are just tender. Season with salt and black pepper.

6. In a separate saucepan, combine crushed tomatoes, minced garlic, dried Italian seasoning, salt, and black pepper. Simmer the tomato sauce over low heat for about 10 minutes, stirring occasionally.

7. Once the turkey meatballs are done, add them to the tomato sauce and simmer for an additional 5 minutes.

8. Serve the Baked Turkey Meatballs over a bed of zucchini noodles, topped with tomato sauce.

9. Enjoy this light and flavorful dish with a sprinkle of additional Parmesan cheese if desired.

Salmon and Vegetable Skewers

Ingredients:

- 1 pound salmon filets, cut into cubes
- 1 red bell pepper, cut into chunks

- 1 yellow bell pepper, cut into chunks
- 1 zucchini, sliced
- 1 red onion, cut into chunks
- Cherry tomatoes
- 2 tablespoons olive oil
- 2 tablespoons fresh lemon juice
- 2 cloves garlic, minced
- 1 teaspoon dried dill
- Salt and black pepper, to taste
- Wooden skewers, soaked in water for 30 minutes

Instructions:

1. Preheat your grill or grill pan to medium-high heat.
2. In a bowl, whisk together olive oil, fresh lemon juice, minced garlic, dried dill, salt, and black pepper.
3. Thread salmon cubes, bell pepper chunks, zucchini slices, red onion chunks, and cherry tomatoes onto the soaked wooden skewers, alternating the ingredients.
4. Brush the skewers with the lemon dill marinade, ensuring they are well coated.

5. Place the skewers on the preheated grill and cook for about 3-4 minutes per side, or until the salmon is cooked through and the vegetables are tender and slightly charred.

6. While grilling, you can baste the skewers with any remaining marinade for extra flavor.

7. Once done, remove the skewers from the grill.

8. Serve the Salmon and Vegetable Skewers on a platter.

9. Optionally, garnish with additional fresh dill and lemon wedges.

10. Enjoy these flavorful and colorful skewers as a healthy and delicious main course.

Lean Turkey Chili

Ingredients:

- 1 pound lean ground turkey
- 1 tablespoon olive oil
- 1 onion, finely chopped
- 3 cloves garlic, minced
- 1 bell pepper, diced
- 1 jalapeño, seeded and finely chopped (optional, for heat)

- 1 can (15 ounces) kidney beans, drained and rinsed
- 1 can (15 ounces) black beans, drained and rinsed
- 1 can (14 ounces) diced tomatoes
- 1 can (6 ounces) tomato paste
- 2 cups low-sodium chicken broth
- 2 teaspoons chili powder
- 1 teaspoon ground cumin
- 1 teaspoon smoked paprika
- 1/2 teaspoon dried oregano
- Salt and black pepper, to taste
- Optional toppings: shredded cheese, chopped green onions, Greek yogurt, cilantro

Instructions:

1. In a large pot or Dutch oven, heat the olive oil over medium heat.
2. Add the ground turkey and cook, breaking it apart with a spoon, until browned and cooked through.

3. Add chopped onion, minced garlic, diced bell pepper, and jalapeño (if using). Cook for an additional 3-4 minutes until the vegetables are softened.

4. Stir in the chili powder, ground cumin, smoked paprika, and dried oregano. Cook for 1-2 minutes to toast the spices.

5. Add the diced tomatoes, tomato paste, kidney beans, black beans, and chicken broth. Season with salt and black pepper to taste.

6. Bring the chili to a boil, then reduce the heat to low, cover, and simmer for at least 30 minutes to allow the flavors to meld. You can simmer longer for deeper flavors.

7. Adjust the seasoning if needed. If the chili is too thick, you can add more chicken broth.

8. Serve the Lean Turkey Chili hot, garnished with your favorite toppings such as shredded cheese, chopped green onions, Greek yogurt, or cilantro.

9. Enjoy your hearty and nutritious Turkey Chili!

Baked Lemon Garlic Tilapia

Ingredients:

- 4 tilapia filets
- 2 tablespoons olive oil
- 3 cloves garlic, minced
- Zest of 1 lemon
- Juice of 1 lemon
- 1 teaspoon dried oregano
- 1 teaspoon dried thyme
- Salt and black pepper, to taste
- Fresh parsley, chopped, for garnish
- Lemon wedges for serving

Instructions:

1. Preheat your oven to 400°F (200°C). Line a baking sheet with parchment paper.
2. Place the tilapia filets on the prepared baking sheet.
3. In a small bowl, whisk together olive oil, minced garlic, lemon zest, lemon juice, dried oregano, dried thyme, salt, and black pepper.
4. Pour the lemon garlic mixture over the tilapia filets, making sure they are well coated on both sides.

5. If you prefer, you can let the tilapia marinate for about 15-30 minutes for additional flavor.

6. Bake in the preheated oven for about 12-15 minutes or until the tilapia is cooked through and easily flakes with a fork.

7. If you desire a golden crust, you can broil the tilapia for an additional 2-3 minutes.

8. Remove the Baked Lemon Garlic Tilapia from the oven, sprinkle with fresh chopped parsley, and serve with lemon wedges on the side.

9. Enjoy this light and delicious Baked Lemon Garlic Tilapia.

Herb-Roasted Chicken Thighs with Sweet Potatoes

Ingredients:

- 4 bone-in, skin-on chicken thighs
- 3 medium sweet potatoes, peeled and cut into chunks
- 3 tablespoons olive oil
- 3 cloves garlic, minced
- 1 teaspoon dried rosemary
- 1 teaspoon dried thyme

- 1 teaspoon dried sage
- Salt and black pepper, to taste
- 1 lemon, sliced
- Fresh parsley, chopped, for garnish

Instructions:

1. Preheat your oven to 425°F (220°C). Line a baking sheet with parchment paper.

2. In a small bowl, mix together olive oil, minced garlic, dried rosemary, dried thyme, dried sage, salt, and black pepper.

3. Place the chicken thighs and sweet potato chunks on the prepared baking sheet.

4. Brush the chicken thighs and sweet potatoes with the herb-infused olive oil mixture, ensuring they are well coated.

5. Place lemon slices on top of the chicken thighs.

6. Roast in the preheated oven for about 35-40 minutes or until the chicken is cooked through and the sweet potatoes are tender, turning the sweet potatoes halfway through.

7. If you desire a golden crust on the chicken, you can broil for an additional 2-3 minutes.

8. Remove the Herb-Roasted Chicken Thighs with Sweet Potatoes from the oven.

9. Garnish with fresh chopped parsley.

10. Serve the chicken thighs and sweet potatoes on a platter, with lemon slices.

11. Enjoy this flavorful and comforting dish for a hearty dinner.

Mango Salsa Chicken

Ingredients:

For the Chicken:

- 4 boneless, skinless chicken breasts
- 1 tablespoon olive oil
- 1 teaspoon ground cumin
- 1 teaspoon chili powder
- Salt and black pepper, to taste

For the Mango Salsa:

- 2 ripe mangoes, peeled, pitted, and diced
- 1/2 red onion, finely chopped
- 1 red bell pepper, diced
- 1 jalapeño, seeded and finely chopped
- 1/4 cup fresh cilantro, chopped
- Juice of 2 limes

- Salt, to taste

Instructions:

1. Preheat your grill or grill pan over medium-high heat.
2. In a small bowl, mix together olive oil, ground cumin, chili powder, salt, and black pepper.
3. Brush the chicken breasts with the spice mixture, ensuring they are well coated on both sides.
4. Grill the chicken breasts for about 6-8 minutes per side or until they are cooked through and have distinct grill marks.
5. While the chicken is grilling, prepare the mango salsa. In a bowl, combine diced mangoes, finely chopped red onion, diced red bell pepper, chopped jalapeño, chopped cilantro, lime juice, and salt. Mix well.
6. Once the chicken is done, remove it from the grill and let it rest for a few minutes.
7. Serve the grilled chicken breasts topped with generous spoonfuls of Mango Salsa.
8. Optionally, garnish with additional cilantro and lime wedges.

9. Enjoy this vibrant and flavorful Mango Salsa Chicken.

Lemon Dill Grilled Shrimp

Ingredients:

- 1 pound large shrimp, peeled and deveined
- 2 tablespoons olive oil
- Zest of 1 lemon
- Juice of 1 lemon
- 2 cloves garlic, minced
- 1 tablespoon fresh dill, chopped
- Salt and black pepper, to taste
- Lemon wedges, for serving

Instructions:

1. Preheat your grill or grill pan over medium-high heat.
2. In a bowl, whisk together olive oil, lemon zest, lemon juice, minced garlic, chopped fresh dill, salt, and black pepper.
3. Place the peeled and deveined shrimp in a shallow dish and pour the lemon dill marinade over them.

4. Toss to coat the shrimp evenly. Allow them to marinate for about 15-30 minutes.

5. Thread the marinated shrimp onto skewers, ensuring they are evenly distributed.

6. Grill the shrimp skewers for about 2-3 minutes per side or until they turn pink and opaque. Be cautious not to overcook, as shrimp cook quickly.

7. While grilling, you can baste the shrimp with any remaining marinade for extra flavor.

8. Once done, remove the shrimp skewers from the grill.

9. Serve the Lemon Dill Grilled Shrimp hot, with lemon wedges on the side.

10. Enjoy this light and zesty grilled shrimp as a delightful appetizer or main dish.

Baked Herb-Crusted Cod

Ingredients:

- 4 cod filets (about 6 ounces each)
- 2 tablespoons olive oil
- 1 cup breadcrumbs (you can use panko for extra crispiness)

- 2 tablespoons fresh parsley, chopped
- 1 teaspoon dried thyme
- 1 teaspoon dried oregano
- 1 teaspoon garlic powder
- Salt and black pepper, to taste
- Lemon wedges, for serving

Instructions:

1. Preheat your oven to 400°F (200°C). Line a baking sheet with parchment paper.
2. In a shallow dish, combine breadcrumbs, chopped fresh parsley, dried thyme, dried oregano, garlic powder, salt, and black pepper.
3. Brush each cod filet with olive oil, ensuring they are well coated.
4. Dip each cod filet into the breadcrumb mixture, pressing the crumbs onto the fish to adhere.
5. Place the coated cod filets on the prepared baking sheet.
6. Bake in the preheated oven for about 12-15 minutes or until the cod is cooked through and the crust is golden brown.
7. If you desire a more golden crust, you can broil the cod for an additional 2-3 minutes.

8. Remove the Baked Herb-Crusted Cod from the oven.

9. Serve the cod filets hot, with lemon wedges on the side.

10. Enjoy this flavorful and light Baked Herb-Crusted Cod.

Chicken and Vegetable Curry

Ingredients:

- 1.5 pounds boneless, skinless chicken thighs, cut into bite-sized pieces
- 2 tablespoons vegetable oil
- 1 large onion, finely chopped
- 3 cloves garlic, minced
- 1 tablespoon fresh ginger, grated
- 2 tablespoons curry powder
- 1 teaspoon ground cumin
- 1 teaspoon ground coriander
- 1/2 teaspoon turmeric
- 1/2 teaspoon chili powder (adjust to taste for spiciness)
- 1 can (14 ounces) diced tomatoes
- 1 can (14 ounces) coconut milk

- 1 cup chicken broth
- 1 large carrot, sliced
- 1 bell pepper, diced
- 1 zucchini, sliced
- Salt and black pepper, to taste
- Fresh cilantro, chopped, for garnish
- Cooked rice, for serving

Instructions:

1. In a large skillet or Dutch oven, heat the vegetable oil over medium heat.

2. Add chopped onion and sauté until softened, about 3-4 minutes.

3. Add minced garlic and grated ginger, stirring for another 1-2 minutes until fragrant.

4. Add the chicken pieces to the skillet and cook until browned on all sides.

5. Sprinkle curry powder, ground cumin, ground coriander, turmeric, and chili powder over the chicken. Stir well to coat the chicken with the spices.

6. Pour in the diced tomatoes (with their juice), coconut milk, and chicken broth. Bring the mixture to a simmer.

7. Add sliced carrot, diced bell pepper, and sliced zucchini to the curry. Season with salt and black pepper to taste.

8. Simmer the curry for about 20-25 minutes or until the chicken is cooked through and the vegetables are tender.

9. Adjust the seasoning if needed. If you prefer a thicker curry, you can let it simmer for a bit longer.

10. Serve the Chicken and Vegetable Curry over cooked rice.

11. Garnish with chopped fresh cilantro.

12. Enjoy this flavorful and comforting Chicken and Vegetable Curry.

Pork Tenderloin with Apple Cider Glaze

Ingredients:

For the Pork Tenderloin:

- 2 pork tenderloins (about 1 pound each)
- Salt and black pepper, to taste
- 1 tablespoon olive oil

For the Apple Cider Glaze:

- 1 cup apple cider
- 2 tablespoons maple syrup
- 1 tablespoon Dijon mustard
- 1 tablespoon apple cider vinegar
- 1 teaspoon cornstarch (optional, for thickening)

Instructions:

1. Preheat your oven to 375°F (190°C).

2. Season the pork tenderloins with salt and black pepper.

3. In an ovenproof skillet, heat olive oil over medium-high heat.

4. Sear the pork tenderloins on all sides until they develop a golden brown crust.

5. Transfer the skillet to the preheated oven and roast for about 15-20 minutes or until the internal temperature of the pork reaches 145°F (63°C).

6. While the pork is roasting, prepare the Apple Cider Glaze. In a small saucepan, combine apple cider, maple syrup, Dijon mustard, and apple cider vinegar. Bring the mixture to a simmer over medium heat.

7. If you prefer a thicker glaze, you can mix cornstarch with a small amount of water to create a slurry. Add the slurry to the simmering glaze and stir until it thickens. Remove from heat.

8. Once the pork is done, remove it from the oven and let it rest for a few minutes.

9. Slice the pork tenderloins and drizzle the Apple Cider Glaze over the top.

10. Serve the Pork Tenderloin with Apple Cider Glaze with your favorite side dishes.

11. Enjoy this flavorful and elegant pork dish with a touch of sweet and tangy glaze.

CHAPTER 9: VEGETABLE
RECIPES

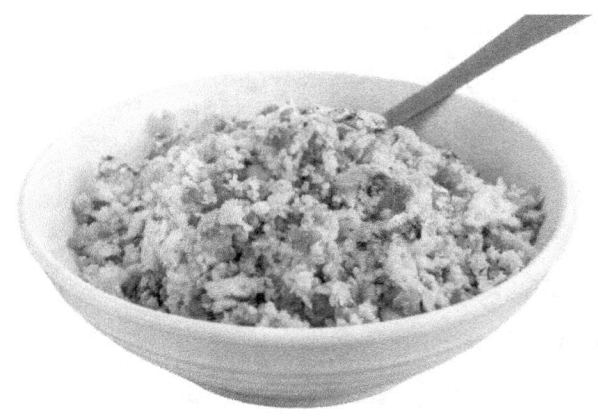

Grilled Zucchini Salad

Ingredients:

For the Grilled Zucchini:

- 3 medium zucchini, sliced lengthwise
- 2 tablespoons olive oil
- Salt and black pepper, to taste
- 1 teaspoon dried oregano
- 1 teaspoon garlic powder

For the Salad:

- 4 cups mixed salad greens
- 1 cup cherry tomatoes, halved

- 1/2 cup feta cheese, crumbled
- 1/4 cup red onion, thinly sliced
- 1/4 cup Kalamata olives, pitted and sliced

For the Dressing:
- 3 tablespoons extra-virgin olive oil
- 1 tablespoon balsamic vinegar
- 1 teaspoon Dijon mustard
- Salt and black pepper, to taste
- Fresh basil, chopped, for garnish

Instructions:

1. Preheat your grill or grill pan over medium-high heat.
2. In a bowl, toss the zucchini slices with olive oil, salt, black pepper, dried oregano, and garlic powder.
3. Grill the zucchini slices for about 2-3 minutes per side, or until they have grill marks and are tender.
4. Remove the grilled zucchini from the heat and let them cool slightly.
5. In a large salad bowl, combine the mixed salad greens, cherry tomatoes, crumbled feta cheese, sliced red onion, and Kalamata olives.

6. Arrange the grilled zucchini slices on top of the salad.

7. In a small bowl, whisk together the extra-virgin olive oil, balsamic vinegar, Dijon mustard, salt, and black pepper to create the dressing.

8. Drizzle the dressing over the Grilled Zucchini Salad.

9. Garnish with fresh chopped basil.

10. Toss the salad gently to combine all the ingredients.

11. Serve immediately and enjoy this light and flavorful Grilled Zucchini Salad.

Roasted Brussels Sprouts with Lemon Garlic Drizzle

Ingredients:
- 1 pound Brussels sprouts, trimmed and halved
- 2 tablespoons olive oil
- Salt and black pepper, to taste
- 2 cloves garlic, minced
- Zest of 1 lemon
- Juice of 1 lemon

- 2 tablespoons grated Parmesan cheese (optional)
- Chopped fresh parsley, for garnish

Instructions:

1. Preheat your oven to 400°F (200°C).
2. In a large bowl, toss the halved Brussels sprouts with olive oil, salt, and black pepper.
3. Spread the Brussels sprouts in a single layer on a baking sheet.
4. Roast in the preheated oven for about 20-25 minutes or until the Brussels sprouts are golden brown and crispy on the edges, tossing halfway through for even cooking.
5. While the Brussels sprouts are roasting, prepare the lemon garlic drizzle. In a small bowl, combine minced garlic, lemon zest, and lemon juice.
6. Once the Brussels sprouts are done, transfer them to a serving dish.
7. Drizzle the lemon garlic mixture over the roasted Brussels sprouts.
8. If desired, sprinkle grated Parmesan cheese over the top.
9. Garnish with chopped fresh parsley.

10. Toss gently to coat the Brussels sprouts with the lemon garlic drizzle.

11. Serve the Roasted Brussels Sprouts with Lemon Garlic Drizzle as a flavorful side dish.

Cauliflower Rice Stir-Fry

Ingredients:

For the Cauliflower Rice:

- 1 large cauliflower head, cleaned and grated (or you can use store-bought cauliflower rice)

For the Stir-Fry:

- 2 tablespoons sesame oil
- 1 pound shrimp, chicken, or tofu, diced (choose based on your preference)
- 1 cup broccoli florets
- 1 bell pepper, thinly sliced
- 1 carrot, julienned
- 1 cup snap peas, trimmed
- 3 green onions, chopped
- 3 cloves garlic, minced
- 1 tablespoon fresh ginger, grated
- 1/4 cup soy sauce
- 2 tablespoons oyster sauce
- 1 tablespoon rice vinegar

- 1 teaspoon Sriracha sauce (optional, for heat)
- Sesame seeds, for garnish
- Chopped cilantro, for garnish

Instructions:

For the Cauliflower Rice:

1. Clean the cauliflower and cut it into florets.
2. Use a food processor or box grater to grate the cauliflower into rice-sized pieces.
3. Place the grated cauliflower in a clean kitchen towel or cheesecloth and squeeze out excess moisture.
4. Set aside the cauliflower rice.

For the Stir-Fry:

1. Heat sesame oil in a large wok or skillet over medium-high heat.
2. Add diced protein (shrimp, chicken, or tofu) to the pan and cook until fully cooked and browned. Remove from the pan and set aside.
3. In the same pan, add a bit more sesame oil if needed. Add minced garlic and grated ginger, sautéing for about 1 minute until fragrant.

4. Add broccoli, bell pepper, julienned carrot, and snap peas to the pan. Stir-fry for 3-4 minutes until the vegetables are slightly tender but still crisp.

5. Push the vegetables to the side of the pan and add the cauliflower rice. Cook for an additional 3-4 minutes, stirring occasionally.

6. Return the cooked protein to the pan.

7. In a small bowl, mix together soy sauce, oyster sauce, rice vinegar, and Sriracha (if using).

8. Pour the sauce over the stir-fry and toss everything together to combine.

9. Cook for an additional 2-3 minutes, ensuring everything is heated through.

10. Garnish with chopped green onions, sesame seeds, and chopped cilantro.

11. Serve the Cauliflower Rice Stir-Fry hot and enjoy this flavorful and low-carb alternative to traditional stir-fry.

Spinach and Mushroom Stuffed Bell Peppers

Ingredients:

- 4 large bell peppers, halved and seeds removed

- 1 tablespoon olive oil
- 1 small onion, finely chopped
- 2 cloves garlic, minced
- 8 ounces mushrooms, finely chopped
- 5 cups fresh spinach, chopped
- 1 cup cooked quinoa or rice
- 1/2 cup grated Parmesan cheese
- Salt and black pepper, to taste
- 1 teaspoon dried oregano
- 1 teaspoon dried thyme
- 1 cup marinara sauce
- 1 cup shredded mozzarella cheese
- Fresh parsley, chopped, for garnish

Instructions:

1. Preheat your oven to 375°F (190°C).
2. Place the bell pepper halves in a baking dish, cut side up.
3. In a large skillet, heat olive oil over medium heat.
4. Add chopped onion and sauté until softened, about 3-4 minutes.
5. Add minced garlic and cook for an additional 1-2 minutes until fragrant.

6. Add chopped mushrooms to the skillet and cook until they release their moisture and become golden brown.

7. Stir in chopped spinach and cook until wilted.

8. In a large mixing bowl, combine the mushroom and spinach mixture with cooked quinoa or rice, grated Parmesan cheese, salt, black pepper, dried oregano, and dried thyme. Mix well.

9. Spoon the stuffing mixture into the halved bell peppers.

10. Pour marinara sauce over the stuffed peppers.

11. Cover the baking dish with foil and bake in the preheated oven for 25-30 minutes or until the peppers are tender.

12. Remove the foil, sprinkle shredded mozzarella cheese over the top of each stuffed pepper, and bake for an additional 10 minutes or until the cheese is melted and bubbly.

13. Garnish with chopped fresh parsley before serving.

14. Serve the Spinach and Mushroom Stuffed Bell Peppers hot, and enjoy this flavorful and nutritious dish.

Asparagus Lemon Basil Quinoa

Ingredients:

- 1 cup quinoa, rinsed
- 2 cups vegetable broth or water
- 1 bunch asparagus, trimmed and cut into bite-sized pieces
- 1 tablespoon olive oil
- Zest of 1 lemon
- Juice of 1 lemon
- 1/4 cup fresh basil, chopped
- Salt and black pepper, to taste
- Grated Parmesan cheese (optional), for serving

Instructions:

1. In a medium saucepan, combine quinoa and vegetable broth (or water). Bring to a boil, then reduce the heat to low, cover, and simmer for about 15 minutes or until the quinoa is cooked and the liquid is absorbed.

2. While the quinoa is cooking, heat olive oil in a large skillet over medium heat.

3. Add the trimmed asparagus pieces to the skillet and sauté for 5-7 minutes or until they are tender-crisp.

4. In a small bowl, whisk together lemon zest, lemon juice, chopped fresh basil, salt, and black pepper.

5. Once the quinoa is cooked, fluff it with a fork and transfer it to a large bowl.

6. Add the sautéed asparagus to the quinoa.

7. Pour the lemon basil dressing over the quinoa and asparagus. Toss everything together until well combined.

8. Season with additional salt and black pepper to taste.

9. Serve the Asparagus Lemon Basil Quinoa warm.

10. Optionally, sprinkle grated Parmesan cheese on top before serving.

11. Enjoy this light and refreshing quinoa dish as a side or a light main course.

Steamed Broccoli with Almond Slivers

Ingredients:

- 1 pound broccoli florets
- 2 tablespoons olive oil
- 2 cloves garlic, minced
- 1/4 cup almond slivers

- Salt and black pepper, to taste
- Lemon wedges, for serving (optional)

Instructions:

1. Bring a pot of water to a boil. Place a steamer basket over the boiling water.
2. Add the broccoli florets to the steamer basket and steam for about 4-5 minutes or until the broccoli is tender but still crisp.
3. While the broccoli is steaming, heat olive oil in a small skillet over medium heat.
4. Add minced garlic to the skillet and sauté for 1-2 minutes until fragrant. Be careful not to let it brown.
5. Add almond slivers to the skillet and toast them for about 2-3 minutes, stirring frequently until they are golden brown.
6. Once the broccoli is steamed, transfer it to a serving dish.
7. Pour the garlic and almond mixture over the steamed broccoli.
8. Season with salt and black pepper to taste.
9. Toss the broccoli and almonds together until well coated.

10. Optionally, squeeze lemon wedges over the top before serving for added freshness.

11. Serve the Steamed Broccoli with Almond Slivers as a delicious and nutritious side dish.

Sautéed Kale with Garlic and Cherry Tomatoes

Ingredients:

- 1 bunch kale, stems removed and leaves chopped
- 2 tablespoons olive oil
- 3 cloves garlic, minced
- 1 pint cherry tomatoes, halved
- Salt and black pepper, to taste
- Crushed red pepper flakes (optional, for heat)
- Lemon wedges, for serving

Instructions:

1. In a large skillet, heat olive oil over medium heat.

2. Add minced garlic to the skillet and sauté for 1-2 minutes until fragrant, being careful not to let it brown.

3. Add the chopped kale to the skillet and toss to coat it in the garlic-infused oil.

4. Sauté the kale for 3-5 minutes or until it wilts and becomes tender.

5. Add halved cherry tomatoes to the skillet and continue to sauté for an additional 2-3 minutes until the tomatoes soften and release their juices.

6. Season the sautéed kale and tomatoes with salt and black pepper to taste.

7. If you like some heat, you can add crushed red pepper flakes to the skillet.

8. Toss everything together until well combined.

9. Once the kale is tender and the tomatoes are cooked, remove the skillet from the heat.

10. Serve the Sautéed Kale with Garlic and Cherry Tomatoes hot, with lemon wedges on the side for squeezing over the top.

11. Enjoy this vibrant and nutritious side dish.

Eggplant and Tomato Bake

Ingredients:

- 2 medium-sized eggplants, sliced into 1/2-inch rounds

- 2 tablespoons olive oil

- Salt and black pepper, to taste

- 1 onion, finely chopped

- 3 cloves garlic, minced

- 1 can (14 ounces) diced tomatoes, drained

- 1 teaspoon dried oregano

- 1 teaspoon dried basil

- 1/2 teaspoon dried thyme

- 1/4 teaspoon red pepper flakes (optional, for heat)

- 1 cup shredded mozzarella cheese

- 1/4 cup grated Parmesan cheese

- Fresh basil, chopped, for garnish (optional)

Instructions:

1. Preheat your oven to 375°F (190°C).

2. Place the eggplant slices on a baking sheet. Brush both sides of each slice with olive oil and season with salt and black pepper.

3. Bake the eggplant slices in the preheated oven for about 15-20 minutes or until they are tender and slightly golden brown. Remove from the oven and set aside.

4. In a skillet, heat a bit of olive oil over medium heat. Add chopped onion and sauté until softened, about 3-4 minutes.

5. Add minced garlic to the skillet and cook for an additional 1-2 minutes until fragrant.

6. Stir in diced tomatoes, dried oregano, dried basil, dried thyme, and red pepper flakes (if using). Cook for about 5 minutes until the mixture thickens slightly.

7. In a baking dish, layer half of the eggplant slices. Spoon half of the tomato mixture over the eggplant.

8. Sprinkle half of the mozzarella and Parmesan cheese over the tomato mixture.

9. Repeat the layers with the remaining eggplant, tomato mixture, and cheeses.

10. Bake in the oven for about 20-25 minutes or until the cheese is melted and bubbly.

11. Remove from the oven and let it cool for a few minutes.

12. Garnish with fresh chopped basil if desired.

13. Serve the Eggplant and Tomato Bake as a delicious and hearty side dish.

Cabbage and Carrot Slaw

Ingredients:

For the Slaw:

- 4 cups shredded green cabbage
- 1 cup shredded carrots
- 1/2 cup thinly sliced red onion
- 1/4 cup chopped fresh cilantro or parsley (optional)

For the Dressing:

- 1/4 cup mayonnaise
- 2 tablespoons apple cider vinegar
- 1 tablespoon Dijon mustard
- 1 tablespoon honey or maple syrup
- Salt and black pepper, to taste

Instructions:

1. In a large bowl, combine shredded green cabbage, shredded carrots, sliced red onion, and chopped cilantro or parsley.

2. In a small bowl, whisk together mayonnaise, apple cider vinegar, Dijon mustard, honey or maple syrup, salt, and black pepper. Adjust the sweetness and acidity to your liking.

3. Pour the dressing over the cabbage and carrot mixture.

4. Toss everything together until the vegetables are well coated with the dressing.

5. Refrigerate the slaw for at least 30 minutes before serving to allow the flavors to meld.

6. Before serving, toss the slaw again to ensure an even coating of dressing.

7. Serve the Cabbage and Carrot Slaw as a refreshing side dish.

Mushroom and Spinach Quiche with Sweet Potato Crust

Ingredients:

For the Sweet Potato Crust:

- 2 medium sweet potatoes, peeled and grated
- 2 tablespoons olive oil
- Salt and black pepper, to taste

For the Quiche Filling:

- 1 tablespoon olive oil
- 1 small onion, finely chopped
- 8 ounces mushrooms, sliced
- 3 cups fresh spinach, chopped

- 4 large eggs
- 1 cup milk (dairy or plant-based)
- Salt and black pepper, to taste
- 1/2 teaspoon dried thyme
- 1/2 cup shredded cheese (cheddar, Swiss, or your choice)

Instructions:

For the Sweet Potato Crust:

1. Preheat your oven to 375°F (190°C).
2. In a bowl, combine grated sweet potatoes with olive oil, salt, and black pepper.
3. Press the sweet potato mixture into the base and sides of a pie dish to form the crust.
4. Bake the sweet potato crust in the preheated oven for about 15-20 minutes or until the edges are golden brown.
5. Remove from the oven and set aside.

For the Quiche Filling:

1. In a skillet, heat olive oil over medium heat.
2. Add chopped onion and sauté until softened, about 3-4 minutes.

3. Add sliced mushrooms to the skillet and cook until they release their moisture and become golden brown.

4. Stir in chopped spinach and cook until wilted. Remove from heat.

5. In a bowl, whisk together eggs, milk, salt, black pepper, and dried thyme.

6. Spread the mushroom and spinach mixture over the sweet potato crust in the pie dish.

7. Pour the egg mixture over the vegetables.

8. Sprinkle shredded cheese on top.

9. Bake the quiche in the oven for 30-35 minutes or until the filling is set and the top is golden brown.

10. Remove from the oven and let it cool for a few minutes before slicing.

11. Serve the Mushroom and Spinach Quiche with Sweet Potato Crust warm.

Stir-Fried Bok Choy with Ginger

Ingredients:

- 2 bunches baby bok choy, cleaned and halved
- 2 tablespoons vegetable oil

- 2 cloves garlic, minced
- 1 tablespoon fresh ginger, grated
- 2 tablespoons soy sauce
- 1 tablespoon oyster sauce
- 1 teaspoon sesame oil
- 1 teaspoon sugar
- Sesame seeds, for garnish (optional)
- Green onions, sliced, for garnish (optional)

Instructions:

1. Trim the ends of the baby bok choy and cut them in half lengthwise.
2. In a small bowl, mix together soy sauce, oyster sauce, sesame oil, and sugar. Set aside.
3. Heat vegetable oil in a wok or large skillet over medium-high heat.
4. Add minced garlic and grated ginger to the hot oil. Stir-fry for about 30 seconds until fragrant.
5. Add the halved baby bok choy to the wok. Stir-fry for 2-3 minutes, tossing the bok choy until it starts to wilt but is still crisp.
6. Pour the sauce mixture over the bok choy.

7. Continue to stir-fry for an additional 1-2 minutes until the bok choy is well coated in the sauce and cooked to your liking.

8. Remove from heat.

9. Garnish with sesame seeds and sliced green onions, if desired.

10. Serve the Stir-Fried Bok Choy with Ginger as a delicious and nutritious side dish.

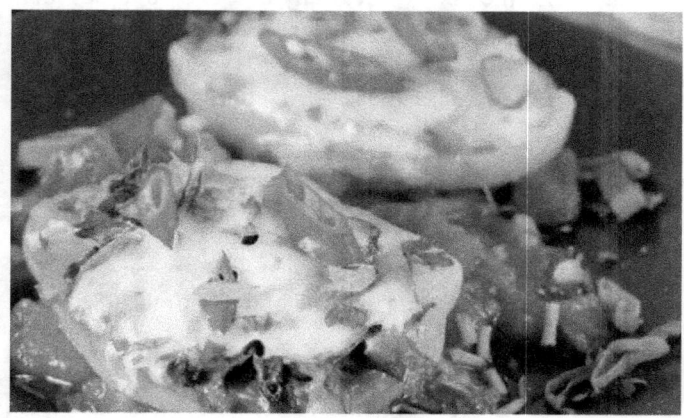

CHAPTER 10: SOUP RECIPES

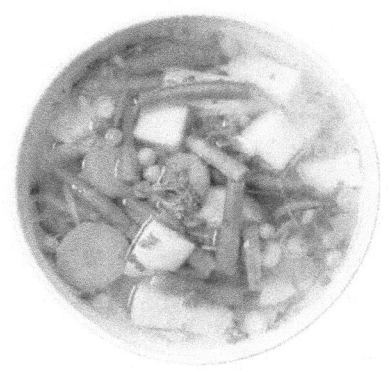

Vegetable Broth Soup

Ingredients:

- 8 cups vegetable broth
- 2 carrots, diced
- 2 celery stalks, diced
- 1 onion, diced
- 2 cloves garlic, minced
- 1 cup diced potatoes
- 1 cup chopped broccoli
- 1 cup chopped cauliflower
- 1 cup sliced mushrooms
- 1 bay leaf
- 1 tsp dried thyme

- Salt and pepper to taste
- Olive oil for sautéing

Instructions:

1. Heat a large pot over medium heat and add a bit of olive oil.
2. Sauté the onion and garlic until translucent.
3. Add carrots and celery, and sauté for a few more minutes.
4. Pour in the vegetable broth and add the bay leaf and dried thyme.
5. Bring the mixture to a boil, then reduce heat to a simmer.
6. Add potatoes, broccoli, cauliflower, and mushrooms. Let simmer for about 15-20 minutes until the vegetables are tender.
7. Remove the bay leaf and season with salt and pepper to taste.
8. Serve hot and enjoy your homemade vegetable broth soup!

Lentil Soup

Ingredients:

- 1 cup dried green or brown lentils, rinsed and drained

- 1 onion, finely chopped
- 2 carrots, diced
- 2 celery stalks, diced
- 3 cloves garlic, minced
- 1 can (14 oz) diced tomatoes
- 6 cups vegetable broth
- 1 tsp ground cumin
- 1 tsp ground coriander
- 1/2 tsp smoked paprika
- 1 bay leaf
- Salt and pepper to taste
- Olive oil for sautéing
- Fresh lemon juice (optional, for serving)

Instructions:

1. Heat a large pot over medium heat and add a bit of olive oil.
2. Sauté the onion, carrots, celery, and garlic until they start to soften, about 5 minutes.
3. Stir in the ground cumin, ground coriander, and smoked paprika, and cook for another 2 minutes to release their flavors.
4. Add the lentils, diced tomatoes (with their juice), vegetable broth, and bay leaf to the pot. Stir well.

5. Bring the mixture to a boil, then reduce heat to a simmer. Cover and let it simmer for about 25-30 minutes, or until the lentils are tender.

6. Remove the bay leaf and season with salt and pepper to taste.

7. If desired, squeeze fresh lemon juice into the soup before serving for a burst of flavor.

8. Serve hot and enjoy your homemade lentil soup!

Tomato Basil Soup

Ingredients:

- 1 can (28 oz) crushed tomatoes
- 1/4 cup olive oil
- 1 small onion, chopped
- 2 cloves garlic, minced
- 1/2 cup fresh basil leaves, chopped
- 2 cups vegetable broth
- Salt and pepper to taste
- 1/2 cup heavy cream (optional for a creamy version)

Instructions:

1. Heat the olive oil in a large pot over medium heat. Add the chopped onion and cook until it becomes translucent, about 5 minutes.

2. Add the minced garlic and cook for another minute until fragrant.

3. Pour in the crushed tomatoes and vegetable broth. Stir well and bring the mixture to a simmer.

4. Add the chopped basil leaves and season with salt and pepper to taste. Let the soup simmer for about 15-20 minutes, allowing the flavors to meld.

5. If you want a creamy version, stir in the heavy cream at this stage. Simmer for an additional 5 minutes.

6. Use an immersion blender to puree the soup until smooth. Alternatively, transfer the soup to a blender in batches, but be cautious as hot liquids can splatter.

7. Return the soup to the pot and heat it through. Taste and adjust the seasoning if needed.

8. Serve hot, garnished with additional fresh basil leaves if desired. Enjoy your homemade Tomato Basil Soup!

Minestrone Soup

Ingredients:

- 2 tablespoons olive oil
- 1 onion, chopped
- 2 cloves garlic, minced
- 2 carrots, diced
- 2 celery stalks, diced
- 1 zucchini, diced
- 1 cup green beans, cut into bite-sized pieces
- 1 can (14 oz) diced tomatoes
- 1 can (14 oz) kidney beans, drained and rinsed
- 1 can (14 oz) cannellini beans, drained and rinsed
- 6 cups vegetable broth
- 1 cup small pasta (e.g., ditalini or elbow macaroni)
- 1 teaspoon dried oregano
- 1 teaspoon dried basil
- Salt and pepper to taste
- Grated Parmesan cheese (optional, for garnish)
- Fresh basil leaves (optional, for garnish)

Instructions:

1. Heat the olive oil in a large pot over medium heat. Add the chopped onion, garlic, carrots, and celery. Sauté for about 5 minutes until they begin to soften.

2. Stir in the diced zucchini and green beans and cook for another 3-4 minutes.

3. Add the diced tomatoes (with their juice), kidney beans, cannellini beans, vegetable broth, dried oregano, and dried basil. Stir well.

4. Bring the mixture to a boil, then reduce the heat to a simmer. Cover and let it simmer for about 20 minutes.

5. In a separate pot, cook the small pasta according to the package instructions. Drain and set aside.

6. Once the vegetables in the soup are tender, stir in the cooked pasta.

7. Season the soup with salt and pepper to taste. Adjust the seasoning as needed.

8. Serve hot, garnished with grated Parmesan cheese and fresh basil leaves if desired.

Chicken and Vegetable Soup

Ingredients:

- 1 pound boneless, skinless chicken breasts or thighs, cubed
- 2 tablespoons olive oil
- 1 onion, chopped
- 2 carrots, sliced
- 2 celery stalks, sliced
- 2 cloves garlic, minced
- 6 cups chicken broth
- 1 bay leaf
- 1 teaspoon dried thyme
- Salt and pepper to taste
- 1 cup diced potatoes
- 1 cup diced zucchini
- 1 cup frozen peas
- 1 cup corn kernels (fresh, frozen, or canned)
- Fresh parsley, chopped for garnish (optional)

Instructions:

1. Heat olive oil in a large pot over medium heat. Add the chopped onion, carrots, celery, and garlic. Sauté for about 5 minutes until they start to soften.

2. Add the cubed chicken to the pot and cook until it's no longer pink on the outside.

3. Pour in the chicken broth and add the bay leaf and dried thyme. Season with salt and pepper to taste.

4. Bring the soup to a boil, then reduce the heat to a simmer. Cover and let it simmer for about 15-20 minutes until the chicken is cooked through.

5. Add the diced potatoes and continue to simmer for another 10 minutes or until the potatoes are tender.

6. Stir in the diced zucchini, frozen peas, and corn kernels. Simmer for an additional 5-7 minutes until the vegetables are cooked to your liking.

7. Taste and adjust the seasoning with salt and pepper if needed.

8. Remove the bay leaf, ladle the soup into bowls, and garnish with fresh chopped parsley if desired.

Butternut Squash Soup

Ingredients:

- 1 butternut squash (about 2-3 pounds), peeled, seeded, and diced
- 1 onion, chopped
- 2 carrots, chopped
- 2 celery stalks, chopped
- 2 cloves garlic, minced
- 4 cups vegetable broth
- 1 teaspoon ground cinnamon
- 1/2 teaspoon ground nutmeg
- Salt and pepper to taste
- 2 tablespoons olive oil
- Optional toppings: sour cream, croutons, chopped chives, or roasted pumpkin seeds

Instructions:

1. In a large pot, heat the olive oil over medium heat. Add the chopped onion, carrots, celery, and garlic. Sauté for about 5 minutes until they start to soften.
2. Add the diced butternut squash to the pot.
3. Pour in the vegetable broth, ground cinnamon, and ground nutmeg. Season with salt and pepper to taste.

4. Bring the mixture to a boil, then reduce the heat to a simmer. Cover and let it simmer for about 20-25 minutes, or until the butternut squash is tender when pierced with a fork.

5. Remove the pot from heat. Use an immersion blender to carefully blend the soup until it's smooth and creamy. If you don't have an immersion blender, you can transfer the soup in batches to a regular blender, blend, and return it to the pot.

6. Taste and adjust the seasoning with salt and pepper if needed.

7. Return the pot to low heat and simmer for an additional 5 minutes to heat through.

8. Serve hot, garnished with your choice of toppings like sour cream, croutons, chopped chives, or roasted pumpkin seeds.

Spinach and White Bean Soup

Ingredients:
- 2 tablespoons olive oil
- 1 onion, chopped
- 2 cloves garlic, minced
- 2 carrots, diced

- 2 celery stalks, diced
- 1 can (14 oz) white beans (cannellini or Great Northern), drained and rinsed
- 4 cups vegetable broth egg
- 1 can (14 oz) diced tomatoes
- 1 teaspoon dried thyme
- 1 teaspoon dried rosemary
- Salt and pepper to taste
- 4 cups fresh spinach leaves
- Grated Parmesan cheese for garnish (optional)

Instructions:

1. In a large pot, heat the olive oil over medium heat. Add the chopped onion, garlic, carrots, and celery. Sauté for about 5 minutes until they start to soften.

2. Stir in the white beans, vegetable broth, diced tomatoes (with their juice), dried thyme, dried rosemary, salt, and pepper. Bring the mixture to a boil.

3. Reduce the heat to a simmer, cover the pot, and let it cook for about 15-20 minutes, allowing the flavors to meld together.

4. Stir in the fresh spinach leaves and let them wilt into the soup, which should only take a couple of minutes.

5. Taste and adjust the seasoning with salt and pepper if needed.

6. Serve hot, garnished with grated Parmesan cheese if desired.

Mushroom Barley Soup

Ingredients:

- 1 cup pearl barley
- 2 tablespoons olive oil
- 1 onion, chopped
- 2 cloves garlic, minced
- 8 ounces mushrooms (any variety you prefer), sliced
- 2 carrots, diced
- 2 celery stalks, diced
- 8 cups vegetable or mushroom broth
- 1 teaspoon dried thyme
- 1 bay leaf
- Salt and pepper to taste
- Fresh parsley, chopped for garnish (optional)

Instructions:

1. Rinse the pearl barley under cold water and drain. Set it aside.

2. In a large pot, heat the olive oil over medium heat. Add the chopped onion and garlic. Sauté for about 3-4 minutes until they start to soften.

3. Add the sliced mushrooms to the pot and cook for another 5-7 minutes until they release their moisture and begin to brown.

4. Stir in the diced carrots and celery, and cook for an additional 5 minutes.

5. Pour in the vegetable or mushroom broth and add the pearl barley, dried thyme, bay leaf, salt, and pepper.

6. Bring the mixture to a boil, then reduce the heat to a simmer. Cover and let it cook for about 45-50 minutes, or until the barley is tender and the soup has thickened.

7. Remove the bay leaf and taste the soup. Adjust the seasoning with more salt and pepper if needed.

8. Serve hot, garnished with fresh chopped parsley if desired.

Cabbage Soup

Ingredients:

- 1 tablespoon olive oil
- 1 onion, chopped
- 2 carrots, sliced
- 2 celery stalks, sliced
- 2 cloves garlic, minced
- 1 small head of cabbage, chopped
- 1 can (14 oz) diced tomatoes
- 6 cups vegetable or chicken broth
- 1 teaspoon dried thyme
- 1 bay leaf
- Salt and pepper to taste
- Optional: 1 cup diced potatoes or white beans for added thickness and protein
- Fresh parsley, chopped for garnish (optional)

Instructions:

1. Heat the olive oil in a large pot over medium heat. Add the chopped onion, carrots, celery, and garlic. Sauté for about 5 minutes until they start to soften.
2. Stir in the chopped cabbage and cook for another 5 minutes, allowing it to wilt slightly.

3. Add the diced tomatoes (with their juice), vegetable or chicken broth, dried thyme, bay leaf, salt, and pepper to the pot.
4. If you'd like a heartier soup, you can add diced potatoes or white beans at this point.
5. Bring the mixture to a boil, then reduce the heat to a simmer. Cover and let it cook for about 20-25 minutes, or until the vegetables are tender.
6. Remove the bay leaf and taste the soup. Adjust the seasoning with more salt and pepper if needed.
7. Serve hot, garnished with fresh chopped parsley if desired.

Thai Coconut Soup

Ingredients:
- 1 tablespoon vegetable oil
- 1 small onion, finely chopped
- 2 cloves garlic, minced
- 1-2 red or green Thai chili peppers, thinly sliced (adjust to your spice preference)
- 1-inch piece of fresh ginger, grated
- 2 lemongrass stalks, cut into 2-inch pieces and smashed

- 3 cups chicken or vegetable broth
- 1 can (14 oz) coconut milk
- 2 tablespoons fish sauce (or soy sauce for a vegetarian version)
- 1 tablespoon brown sugar
- 1 cup sliced mushrooms (shiitake or button mushrooms work well)
- 1 cup thinly sliced bell peppers (red or green)
- 1 cup sliced cooked chicken (optional)
- Juice of 1-2 limes, to taste
- Fresh cilantro leaves for garnish
- Fresh Thai basil leaves for garnish (optional)

Instructions:

1. In a large pot, heat the vegetable oil over medium heat. Add the chopped onion, garlic, and Thai chili peppers. Sauté for about 2-3 minutes until fragrant.
2. Stir in the grated ginger and smashed lemongrass stalks and continue to sauté for another 2-3 minutes.
3. Pour in the chicken or vegetable broth and bring it to a simmer. Let it simmer for about 10 minutes to infuse the flavors.
4. Remove and discard the lemongrass stalks.

5. Add the coconut milk, fish sauce (or soy sauce), and brown sugar to the pot. Stir well to combine.

6. Add the sliced mushrooms, bell peppers, and cooked chicken (if using). Let the soup simmer for another 5-7 minutes, or until the vegetables are tender.

7. Stir in the lime juice to taste. Adjust the fish sauce, sugar, or lime juice according to your preference for a balance of sweet, sour, and salty flavors.

8. Serve hot, garnished with fresh cilantro leaves and Thai basil if available.

Fish Chowder

Ingredients:

- 2 tablespoons butter
- 1 onion, chopped
- 2 celery stalks, diced
- 2 carrots, diced
- 2 cloves garlic, minced
- 2 potatoes, peeled and diced
- 4 cups fish or seafood broth
- 1 bay leaf
- 1 teaspoon dried thyme

- 1/2 teaspoon paprika
- Salt and pepper to taste
- 1 cup whole milk or half-and-half
- 1 pound white fish filets (such as cod or haddock), cut into chunks
- 1 cup corn kernels (fresh, frozen, or canned)
- Chopped fresh parsley for garnish

Instructions:

1. In a large pot, melt the butter over medium heat. Add the chopped onion, celery, carrots, and garlic. Sauté for about 5 minutes until they start to soften.

2. Stir in the diced potatoes, fish or seafood broth, bay leaf, dried thyme, paprika, salt, and pepper. Bring the mixture to a boil, then reduce the heat to a simmer. Cover and let it simmer for about 15-20 minutes, or until the potatoes are tender.

3. Remove and discard the bay leaf.

4. Stir in the whole milk or half-and-half.

5. Gently add the chunks of white fish and corn kernels to the pot. Let them simmer for about 5-7 minutes until the fish is cooked through and flakes easily with a fork.

6. Taste and adjust the seasoning with salt and pepper if needed.

7. Serve hot, garnished with chopped fresh parsley.

Broccoli and Cheddar Soup

Ingredients:

- 1 lb fresh broccoli, chopped
- 1 small onion, diced
- 2 carrots, peeled and sliced
- 2 cloves garlic, minced
- 4 cups chicken or vegetable broth
- 1 cup milk
- 1/2 cup heavy cream
- 2 cups shredded cheddar cheese
- 3 tbsp butter
- 3 tbsp all-purpose flour
- Salt and pepper to taste

Instructions:

1. In a large pot, melt butter over medium heat. Add onions and garlic, sauté until softened.

2. Stir in flour to create a roux, cook for 2-3 minutes.

3. Slowly whisk in the broth, followed by the milk and heavy cream. Allow it to simmer.

4. Add chopped broccoli and carrots. Cook until vegetables are tender, about 15-20 minutes.

5. Using an immersion blender, blend the soup until desired consistency is reached.

6. Stir in shredded cheddar cheese until melted. Season with salt and pepper to taste.

7. Serve hot and enjoy your homemade Broccoli and Cheddar Soup!

Spinach and Lentil Soup

Ingredients:

- 1 cup dried green or brown lentils, rinsed and drained
- 2 tablespoons olive oil
- 1 onion, chopped
- 2 carrots, diced
- 2 celery stalks, diced
- 3 cloves garlic, minced
- 6 cups vegetable broth
- 1 can (14 oz) diced tomatoes
- 1 teaspoon ground cumin

- 1 teaspoon ground coriander
- 1/2 teaspoon smoked paprika
- 1 bay leaf
- Salt and pepper to taste
- 4 cups fresh spinach leaves
- Juice of 1-2 lemons, to taste
- Fresh parsley, chopped for garnish (optional)

Instructions:

1. In a large pot, heat the olive oil over medium heat. Add the chopped onion, carrots, celery, and garlic. Sauté for about 5 minutes until they start to soften.

2. Stir in the rinsed lentils, vegetable broth, diced tomatoes (with their juice), ground cumin, ground coriander, smoked paprika, bay leaf, salt, and pepper.

3. Bring the mixture to a boil, then reduce the heat to a simmer. Cover and let it simmer for about 20-25 minutes, or until the lentils are tender.

4. Remove and discard the bay leaf.

5. Stir in the fresh spinach leaves and let them wilt into the soup, which should only take a couple of minutes.

6. Add the lemon juice to taste. Adjust the seasoning with salt, pepper, or more lemon juice if needed.
7. Serve hot, garnished with fresh chopped parsley if desired.

Black Bean Soup

Ingredients:

- 2 tablespoons olive oil
- 1 onion, chopped
- 2 cloves garlic, minced
- 2 carrots, diced
- 2 celery stalks, diced
- 2 red bell peppers, diced
- 2 cans (15 oz each) black beans, drained and rinsed
- 1 can (14 oz) diced tomatoes
- 4 cups vegetable or chicken broth
- 1 teaspoon ground cumin
- 1 teaspoon chili powder
- 1/2 teaspoon smoked paprika
- Salt and pepper to taste
- Juice of 1 lime
- Fresh cilantro, chopped for garnish

- Sour cream or Greek yogurt for garnish (optional)

Instructions:

1. In a large pot, heat the olive oil over medium heat. Add the chopped onion and garlic. Sauté for about 3-4 minutes until they become translucent.

2. Stir in the diced carrots, celery, and red bell peppers. Sauté for another 5 minutes until the vegetables start to soften.

3. Add the drained and rinsed black beans, diced tomatoes (with their juice), vegetable or chicken broth, ground cumin, chili powder, smoked paprika, salt, and pepper to the pot.

4. Bring the mixture to a boil, then reduce the heat to a simmer. Cover and let it simmer for about 20-25 minutes to allow the flavors to meld together.

5. Using an immersion blender, carefully blend the soup until it's mostly smooth, leaving some texture for a chunkier soup. If you don't have an immersion blender, you can transfer a portion of the soup to a regular blender, blend, and return it to the pot.

6. Stir in the lime juice to taste. Adjust the seasoning with salt, pepper, or more lime juice if needed.

7. Serve hot, garnished with fresh chopped cilantro and a dollop of sour cream or Greek yogurt if desired.

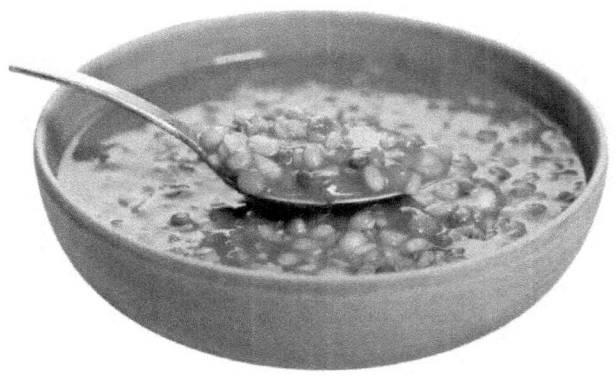

"Optimal liver health is my priority, and I make choices aligned with that goal."

"My body responds positively to the care and nourishment I provide."

CHAPTER 11: SALAD RECIPES

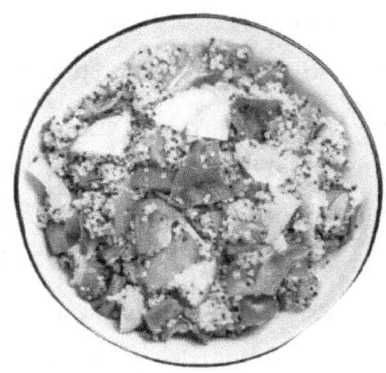

Spinach and Strawberry Salad

Ingredients:

- 6 cups fresh spinach leaves
- 1 1/2 cups sliced strawberries
- 1/4 cup chopped red onion
- 1/4 cup chopped pecans or almonds
- 1/4 cup crumbled feta cheese (optional)
- 2 tablespoons balsamic vinegar
- 2 tablespoons olive oil
- 1 tablespoon honey
- Salt and pepper to taste

Instructions:

1. Wash and dry the spinach leaves thoroughly. Place them in a large salad bowl.
2. Add the sliced strawberries, chopped red onion, and chopped nuts to the bowl.
3. If you're using feta cheese, sprinkle it over the salad.
4. In a small bowl, whisk together the balsamic vinegar, olive oil, honey, salt, and pepper until well combined.
5. Drizzle the dressing over the salad.
6. Toss everything together gently to coat the salad with the dressing.
7. Serve immediately and enjoy your refreshing spinach and strawberry salad!

Mediterranean Quinoa Salad

Ingredients:

For the Salad:

- 1 cup quinoa, rinsed and drained
- 2 cups water
- 1 cup cherry tomatoes, halved
- 1 cucumber, diced
- 1/2 cup red bell pepper, diced

- 1/2 cup green bell pepper, diced
- 1/4 cup red onion, finely chopped
- 1/4 cup Kalamata olives, pitted and sliced
- 1/4 cup fresh parsley, chopped
- 1/4 cup fresh mint, chopped (optional)
- 1/2 cup crumbled feta cheese (optional)

For the Dressing:
- 1/4 cup extra-virgin olive oil
- 2 tablespoons lemon juice
- 2 cloves garlic, minced
- 1 teaspoon dried oregano
- Salt and pepper to taste

Instructions:

1. In a medium saucepan, combine the quinoa and water. Bring to a boil, then reduce the heat to low, cover, and simmer for about 15 minutes, or until the quinoa is cooked and the water is absorbed. Remove from heat and let it cool.

2. In a large salad bowl, combine the cooked and cooled quinoa, cherry tomatoes, cucumber, red and green bell peppers, red onion, Kalamata olives, parsley, and mint (if using).

3. In a small bowl, whisk together the olive oil, lemon juice, minced garlic, dried oregano, salt, and pepper to make the dressing.

4. Pour the dressing over the salad and toss everything together until well combined.

5. If you like, sprinkle crumbled feta cheese over the top of the salad.

6. Chill the Mediterranean Quinoa Salad in the refrigerator for at least 30 minutes before serving to allow the flavors to meld together.

7. Serve as a refreshing and nutritious side dish or a light meal.

Chickpea and Cucumber Salad

Ingredients:

For the Salad:

- 1 can (15 ounces) chickpeas, drained and rinsed
- 1 cucumber, diced
- 1/2 red onion, finely chopped
- 1/2 cup cherry tomatoes, halved
- 1/4 cup fresh parsley, chopped
- 1/4 cup fresh mint, chopped (optional)
- 1/4 cup crumbled feta cheese (optional)

For the Dressing:

- 2 tablespoons extra-virgin olive oil
- 1 tablespoon lemon juice
- 2 cloves garlic, minced
- Salt and pepper to taste

Instructions:

1. In a large salad bowl, combine the chickpeas, diced cucumber, chopped red onion, cherry tomatoes, parsley, and mint (if using).
2. In a small bowl, whisk together the olive oil, lemon juice, minced garlic, salt, and pepper to create the dressing.
3. Pour the dressing over the salad ingredients.
4. Toss everything together until the salad is well coated with the dressing.
5. If desired, sprinkle crumbled feta cheese over the top of the salad.
6. Chill the Chickpea and Cucumber Salad in the refrigerator for about 20-30 minutes to let the flavors meld together.
7. Serve as a light and healthy side dish or enjoy it as a quick and nutritious meal.

Beet and Walnut Salad

Ingredients:

For the Salad:

- 4 medium-sized beets, roasted and peeled
- 1/2 cup walnuts, toasted and roughly chopped
- 1/4 cup crumbled goat cheese (optional)
- 4 cups arugula or mixed greens

For the Dressing:

- 3 tablespoons extra-virgin olive oil
- 2 tablespoons balsamic vinegar
- 1 teaspoon honey
- Salt and pepper to taste

Instructions:

1. Start by roasting the beets. Preheat your oven to 400°F (200°C). Wash the beets and trim off the tops. Wrap each beet in aluminum foil and place them on a baking sheet. Roast for about 45-60 minutes or until they're tender when pierced with a fork. Let them cool, then peel and dice them.

2. While the beets are roasting, toast the walnuts in a dry skillet over medium heat for a few minutes until they become fragrant. Be careful not to burn them. Set aside to cool, then roughly chop.

3. In a small bowl, whisk together the olive oil, balsamic vinegar, honey, salt, and pepper to create the dressing.
4. Place the arugula or mixed greens in a large salad bowl.
5. Add the roasted and diced beets on top of the greens.
6. Sprinkle the toasted and chopped walnuts over the beets.
7. If desired, crumble the goat cheese over the salad.
8. Drizzle the dressing over the salad ingredients.
9. Gently toss everything together to coat the salad with the dressing.
10. Serve your Beet and Walnut Salad as a tasty and colorful appetizer or side dish.

Tuna and White Bean Salad

Ingredients:

For the Salad:

- 2 cans (15 ounces each) white beans (cannellini or Great Northern), drained and rinsed
- 2 cans (5 ounces each) canned tuna in water, drained

- 1/2 red onion, finely chopped
- 1/2 cup cherry tomatoes, halved
- 1/4 cup fresh parsley, chopped
- 1/4 cup pitted black olives, sliced
- 1/4 cup cucumber, diced (optional)
- Salt and pepper to taste

For the Dressing:

- 3 tablespoons extra-virgin olive oil
- 2 tablespoons red wine vinegar
- 1 clove garlic, minced
- 1 teaspoon Dijon mustard
- 1/2 teaspoon dried oregano
- Salt and pepper to taste

Instructions:

1. In a large salad bowl, combine the drained white beans, canned tuna, chopped red onion, halved cherry tomatoes, chopped parsley, olives, and diced cucumber (if using).
2. In a small bowl, whisk together the olive oil, red wine vinegar, minced garlic, Dijon mustard, dried oregano, salt, and pepper to create the dressing.
3. Pour the dressing over the salad ingredients.

4. Gently toss everything together until the salad is well coated with the dressing.

5. Taste and adjust the seasoning with additional salt and pepper if needed.

6. Chill the Tuna and White Bean Salad in the refrigerator for about 20-30 minutes to let the flavors meld together.

7. Serve as a protein-packed and satisfying salad for lunch or dinner.

Broccoli and Cranberry Salad

Ingredients:

For the Salad:

- 4 cups fresh broccoli florets, chopped into bite-sized pieces
- 1/2 cup dried cranberries
- 1/2 cup chopped red onion
- 1/2 cup chopped bacon (cooked and crumbled)
- 1/2 cup chopped pecans or almonds
- 1/2 cup shredded cheddar cheese (optional)

For the Dressing:

- 1/2 cup mayonnaise
- 2 tablespoons white wine vinegar or apple cider vinegar

- 2 tablespoons honey
- Salt and pepper to taste

Instructions:

1. In a large salad bowl, combine the chopped broccoli florets, dried cranberries, chopped red onion, crumbled bacon, chopped nuts, and shredded cheddar cheese (if using).
2. In a separate small bowl, whisk together the mayonnaise, white wine vinegar, honey, salt, and pepper to create the dressing.
3. Pour the dressing over the salad ingredients.
4. Gently toss everything together until the salad is well coated with the dressing.
5. Taste and adjust the seasoning with additional salt and pepper if needed.
6. Chill the Broccoli and Cranberry Salad in the refrigerator for at least 30 minutes before serving to allow the flavors to meld together.
7. Serve as a tasty and colorful side dish at picnics, barbecues, or as a healthy addition to your meals.

Asian Cabbage Salad

Ingredients:

For the Salad:

- 4 cups thinly sliced Napa cabbage (about 1 small head)
- 1 cup shredded carrots
- 1 red bell pepper, thinly sliced
- 1/2 cup chopped scallions (green onions)
- 1/4 cup chopped fresh cilantro
- 1/4 cup chopped fresh mint (optional)
- 1/2 cup chopped roasted peanuts or slivered almonds
- 1/4 cup sesame seeds (toasted, if preferred)
- 1 cup cooked and shredded chicken breast or tofu (optional)

For the Dressing:

- 3 tablespoons soy sauce
- 2 tablespoons rice vinegar
- 2 tablespoons toasted sesame oil
- 1 tablespoon honey or maple syrup
- 1 teaspoon grated fresh ginger
- 1 clove garlic, minced
- Red pepper flakes (optional, for heat)
- Salt and pepper to taste

Instructions:

1. In a large salad bowl, combine the sliced Napa cabbage, shredded carrots, red bell pepper slices, chopped scallions, fresh cilantro, and mint (if using).

2. If you'd like to add protein to your salad, you can include the cooked and shredded chicken breast or tofu.

3. In a separate small bowl, whisk together the soy sauce, rice vinegar, toasted sesame oil, honey or maple syrup, grated ginger, minced garlic, and red pepper flakes (if you want some heat). Season with salt and pepper to taste.

4. Pour the dressing over the salad ingredients.

5. Toss everything together until the salad is well coated with the dressing.

6. Sprinkle the chopped peanuts or slivered almonds and sesame seeds over the top of the salad.

7. Chill the Asian Cabbage Salad in the refrigerator for about 20-30 minutes to allow the flavors to meld together.

8. Serve as a vibrant and satisfying salad, garnished with additional fresh herbs and peanuts if desired.

Caprese Salad

Ingredients:

- 4 large ripe tomatoes, sliced
- 1/4 cup fresh basil leaves
- 8 ounces fresh mozzarella cheese, sliced
- Extra-virgin olive oil, for drizzling
- Balsamic glaze (optional, for drizzling)
- Salt and freshly ground black pepper to taste

Instructions:

1. Begin by washing and slicing the tomatoes into 1/4-inch thick rounds.
2. Slice the fresh mozzarella cheese into rounds that are similar in thickness to the tomatoes.
3. On a serving platter or individual plates, start assembling the salad. Place a tomato slice on the plate, followed by a slice of fresh mozzarella, and then a fresh basil leaf. Repeat this pattern, alternating tomato, mozzarella, and basil until you've used all the slices.

4. Drizzle extra-virgin olive oil evenly over the tomato, mozzarella, and basil stacks. You can also add a few drops of balsamic glaze for extra flavor if you like.

5. Season the Caprese Salad with a pinch of salt and freshly ground black pepper to taste.

6. Serve immediately to enjoy the freshness of this classic Italian salad.

Greek Salad

Ingredients:

For the Salad:

- 4 cups chopped Romaine lettuce or mixed greens
- 1 cucumber, diced
- 1 cup cherry tomatoes, halved
- 1/2 red onion, thinly sliced
- 1/2 cup Kalamata olives, pitted and sliced
- 1/2 cup crumbled feta cheese
- 1/4 cup chopped fresh parsley

For the Dressing:

- 3 tablespoons extra-virgin olive oil
- 2 tablespoons red wine vinegar
- 1 teaspoon dried oregano

- Salt and pepper to taste
- Optional: 1 clove garlic, minced

Instructions:

1. In a large salad bowl, combine the chopped Romaine lettuce or mixed greens, diced cucumber, halved cherry tomatoes, thinly sliced red onion, Kalamata olives, crumbled feta cheese, and chopped fresh parsley.

2. In a small bowl, whisk together the extra-virgin olive oil, red wine vinegar, dried oregano, salt, and pepper. If you like garlic, you can also add minced garlic to the dressing.

3. Pour the dressing over the salad ingredients.

4. Toss everything together gently until the salad is well coated with the dressing.

5. Taste and adjust the seasoning with additional salt and pepper if needed.

6. Serve your Greek Salad as a refreshing and flavorful side dish or add grilled chicken, shrimp, or tofu for a complete meal.

Roasted Vegetable Salad

Ingredients:

For the Roasted Vegetables:

- 2 cups of your choice of vegetables (e.g., bell peppers, zucchini, cherry tomatoes, red onion, carrots, and broccoli), chopped into bite-sized pieces
- 2 tablespoons olive oil
- Salt and pepper to taste
- 1 teaspoon dried herbs (rosemary, thyme, or oregano work well)

For the Salad:

- 4 cups mixed salad greens (e.g., spinach, arugula, or Romaine lettuce)
- 1/2 cup crumbled feta cheese or goat cheese (optional)
- 1/4 cup chopped nuts (e.g., walnuts or almonds)
- Balsamic vinaigrette dressing (store-bought or homemade)

Instructions:

1. Preheat your oven to 425°F (220°C).
2. In a large mixing bowl, toss the chopped vegetables with olive oil, salt, pepper, and dried herbs until they are well coated.

3. Spread the vegetables in a single layer on a baking sheet lined with parchment paper.

4. Roast the vegetables in the preheated oven for 20-25 minutes or until they are tender and slightly caramelized. You may need to stir them once or twice during roasting for even cooking.

5. While the vegetables are roasting, prepare the salad greens in a large serving bowl.

6. Once the roasted vegetables are done, let them cool for a few minutes.

7. Arrange the roasted vegetables on top of the salad greens.

8. If desired, sprinkle crumbled feta cheese or goat cheese and chopped nuts over the top.

9. Drizzle balsamic vinaigrette dressing over the salad, using as much or as little as you like.

10. Toss the salad gently to combine all the ingredients.

11. Serve your Roasted Vegetable Salad as a satisfying and flavorful meal or side dish.

Avocado and Black Bean Salad

Ingredients:

For the Salad:

- 1 can (15 ounces) black beans, drained and rinsed
- 2 ripe avocados, diced
- 1 cup corn kernels (fresh, frozen, or canned)
- 1 cup cherry tomatoes, halved
- 1/4 cup red onion, finely chopped
- 1/4 cup fresh cilantro, chopped
- 1 jalapeño pepper, seeded and finely chopped (optional for heat)
- Juice of 2 limes
- Salt and pepper to taste

For the Dressing:

- 3 tablespoons extra-virgin olive oil
- 1 tablespoon red wine vinegar
- 1 clove garlic, minced
- 1 teaspoon ground cumin
- Salt and pepper to taste

Instructions:

1. In a large salad bowl, combine the black beans, diced avocados, corn kernels, cherry tomatoes, chopped red onion, chopped cilantro, and chopped jalapeño pepper (if using).

2. Squeeze the juice of two limes over the salad ingredients.

3. In a separate small bowl, whisk together the extra-virgin olive oil, red wine vinegar, minced garlic, ground cumin, salt, and pepper to create the dressing.

4. Pour the dressing over the salad ingredients.

5. Gently toss everything together until the salad is well coated with the dressing.

6. Taste and adjust the seasoning with additional salt, pepper, or lime juice if needed.

7. Chill the Avocado and Black Bean Salad in the refrigerator for about 20-30 minutes to allow the flavors to meld together.

8. Serve as a refreshing and nutritious salad, as a side dish, or with tortilla chips as a dip.

Quinoa and Kale Salad

Ingredients:

For the Salad:

- 1 cup quinoa, rinsed and drained
- 2 cups water
- 4 cups kale, stems removed and chopped into bite-sized pieces
- 1 cup cherry tomatoes, halved
- 1 cucumber, diced
- 1/4 cup red onion, finely chopped
- 1/4 cup crumbled feta cheese (optional)
- 1/4 cup chopped almonds or walnuts (toasted, if desired)

For the Dressing:

- 3 tablespoons extra-virgin olive oil
- 2 tablespoons lemon juice
- 2 cloves garlic, minced
- 1 teaspoon Dijon mustard
- Salt and pepper to taste

Instructions:

1. In a medium saucepan, combine the quinoa and water.

2. Bring to a boil, then reduce the heat to low, cover, and simmer for about 15 minutes, or until the quinoa is cooked and the water is absorbed. Remove from heat and let it cool.

3. While the quinoa is cooking, prepare the kale by removing the tough stems and chopping the leaves into bite-sized pieces. Massage the kale leaves with a bit of olive oil to help soften them.

4. In a large salad bowl, combine the cooked and cooled quinoa, chopped kale, halved cherry tomatoes, diced cucumber, and finely chopped red onion.

5. If you're using feta cheese, sprinkle it over the salad.

6. In a small bowl, whisk together the extra-virgin olive oil, lemon juice, minced garlic, Dijon mustard, salt, and pepper to create the dressing.

7. Pour the dressing over the salad ingredients.

8. Toss everything together gently to coat the salad with the dressing.

9. Sprinkle the chopped almonds or walnuts over the top of the salad.

10. Chill the Quinoa and Kale Salad in the refrigerator for about 20-30 minutes before serving to allow the flavors to meld together.

11. Serve as a nutritious and satisfying salad, either as a side dish or a light meal.

Shrimp and Mango Salad

Ingredients:
For the Salad:
- 1 pound large shrimp, peeled and deveined
- 2 ripe mangoes, peeled, pitted, and diced
- 1 red bell pepper, diced
- 1/4 cup red onion, finely chopped
- 1/4 cup fresh cilantro, chopped
- 1/4 cup fresh mint leaves, chopped (optional)
- Mixed salad greens or arugula for serving

For the Dressing:
- 3 tablespoons extra-virgin olive oil
- 2 tablespoons lime juice
- 1 tablespoon honey
- 1 clove garlic, minced
- Salt and pepper to taste
- Red pepper flakes (optional, for heat)

Instructions:

1. In a large skillet, heat a bit of olive oil over medium-high heat. Add the shrimp and cook for about 2-3 minutes per side or until they turn pink and opaque. Remove from heat and let them cool.

2. In a large salad bowl, combine the diced mangoes, diced red bell pepper, finely chopped red onion, chopped cilantro, and chopped mint leaves (if using).

3. Once the cooked shrimp have cooled, add them to the salad bowl.

4. In a small bowl, whisk together the extra-virgin olive oil, lime juice, honey, minced garlic, salt, pepper, and red pepper flakes (if you want some heat).

5. Drizzle the dressing over the salad ingredients.

6. Gently toss everything together until the salad is well coated with the dressing.

7. Serve the Shrimp and Mango Salad on a bed of mixed salad greens or arugula.

8. Enjoy this tropical-inspired salad as a light and flavorful meal.

Waldorf Salad

Ingredients:

For the Salad:

- 2 cups diced apples (such as Granny Smith or Red Delicious)
- 1 cup diced celery
- 1/2 cup halved red grapes
- 1/2 cup chopped walnuts or pecans
- 1/2 cup raisins or dried cranberries
- 4 cups fresh lettuce leaves (such as iceberg or Romaine), torn into bite-sized pieces

For the Dressing:

- 1/2 cup mayonnaise
- 2 tablespoons lemon juice
- 1 tablespoon honey
- Salt and pepper to taste

Instructions:

1. In a large salad bowl, combine the diced apples, diced celery, halved red grapes, chopped nuts, and raisins or dried cranberries.
2. In a separate small bowl, whisk together the mayonnaise, lemon juice, honey, salt, and pepper to create the dressing.
3. Pour the dressing over the salad ingredients.

4. Toss everything together gently until the salad is well coated with the dressing.

5. Chill the Waldorf Salad in the refrigerator for about 20-30 minutes to let the flavors meld together.

6. Just before serving, arrange the fresh lettuce leaves on a serving platter or individual plates.

7. Spoon the chilled salad mixture over the lettuce.

8. Serve your Waldorf Salad as a delightful and classic side dish or light meal.

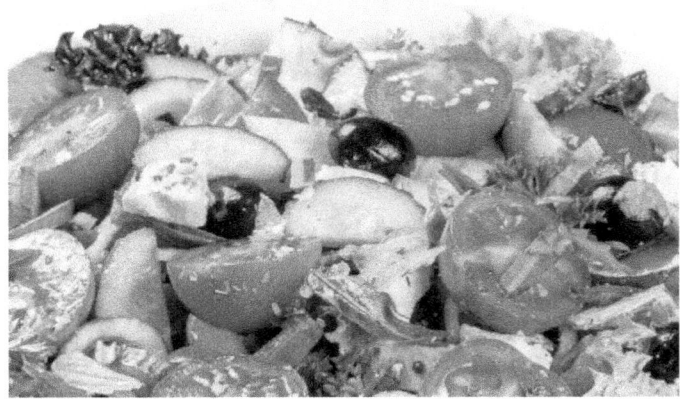

"I am mindful of the foods I consume, promoting liver-friendly choices."

"I am on a path to vibrant health, and my liver is rejuvenating with each healthy choice."

CHAPTER 12: DESSERT RECIPES

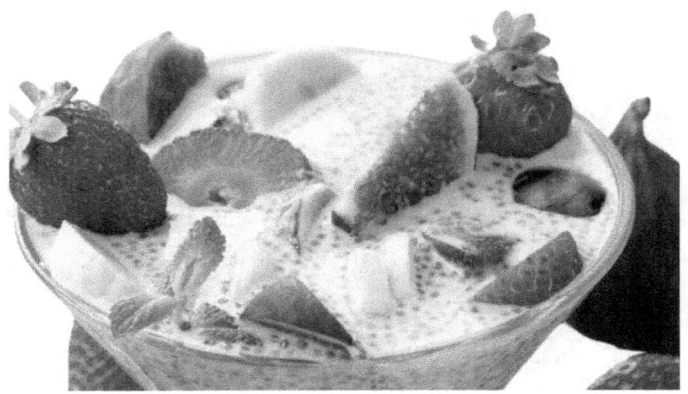

Baked Apples

Ingredients:

- 4 medium-sized apples (such as Granny Smith or Honeycrisp)
- 1/4 cup brown sugar or maple syrup
- 1 teaspoon ground cinnamon
- 1/4 teaspoon ground nutmeg
- 1/4 cup chopped nuts (such as walnuts or pecans)
- 2 tablespoons unsalted butter (or dairy-free alternative)
- 1/2 cup apple juice or apple cider (for baking)

Optional Toppings:

- Vanilla ice cream, whipped cream, or yogurt
- Additional cinnamon and brown sugar for garnish

Instructions:

1. Preheat your oven to 375°F (190°C).
2. Wash and core the apples, leaving the bottoms intact so they can hold the filling. You can use an apple corer or a knife to do this.
3. In a small bowl, mix together the brown sugar, ground cinnamon, ground nutmeg, and chopped nuts.
4. Stuff each cored apple with the sugar and nut mixture, pressing it down slightly.
5. Place a small piece of butter on top of each filled apple.
6. Arrange the stuffed apples in a baking dish with high sides. Pour the apple juice or cider into the bottom of the dish.
7. Cover the baking dish with aluminum foil.
8. Bake the apples in the preheated oven for about 30-40 minutes, or until they are tender. The exact baking time may vary depending on the size and type of apples you use.

9. Once the apples are done, remove them from the oven and allow them to cool slightly.

10. Serve the Baked Apples warm, drizzled with any juices from the baking dish, and topped with a scoop of vanilla ice cream, whipped cream, or yogurt, if desired.

11. For an extra touch of sweetness, sprinkle some additional cinnamon and brown sugar on top before serving.

Berry Parfait

Ingredients:

- 2 cups mixed berries (strawberries, blueberries, raspberries, blackberries, etc.)
- 2 cups Greek yogurt or your favorite yogurt
- 1/4 cup honey or maple syrup (adjust to taste)
- 1 cup granola (homemade or store-bought)
- Fresh mint leaves for garnish (optional)

Instructions:

- Wash and prepare the mixed berries. If using strawberries, remove the stems and slice them.
- In a mixing bowl, combine the Greek yogurt and honey or maple syrup. Stir well to sweeten the yogurt to your liking.

- In serving glasses or bowls, start by layering a spoonful of the sweetened yogurt at the bottom.
- Add a layer of mixed berries on top of the yogurt.
- Sprinkle a layer of granola over the berries.
- Repeat the layers until the glass is filled, finishing with a layer of berries on top.
- Garnish with fresh mint leaves for a pop of color and extra freshness if desired.
- Repeat the layering process for as many parfaits as you'd like to make.
- Serve your Berry Parfaits immediately, or refrigerate them for a refreshing and healthy dessert or breakfast.

Chia Seed Pudding

Ingredients:
- 1/4 cup chia seeds
- 1 cup milk (dairy or dairy-free like almond, coconut, or soy)
- 1-2 tablespoons sweetener (honey, maple syrup, agave nectar, or sugar)
- 1/2 teaspoon vanilla extract (optional)
- A pinch of salt

Toppings (optional):

- Fresh berries, sliced fruits, or fruit compote
- Nuts (e.g., almonds, walnuts)
- Shredded coconut
- Chocolate chips
- Cinnamon or nutmeg
- Yogurt or whipped cream

Instructions:

1. In a mixing bowl, combine the chia seeds, milk, sweetener, vanilla extract (if using), and a pinch of salt.
2. Stir well to mix all the ingredients thoroughly.
3. Cover the bowl and refrigerate for at least 2-3 hours, or overnight if possible. During this time, the chia seeds will absorb the liquid and thicken the pudding.
4. After the pudding has set, give it a good stir to break up any clumps and achieve a creamy consistency.
5. Taste the pudding and adjust the sweetness if needed by adding more sweetener.
6. Divide the Chia Seed Pudding into serving cups or bowls.

7. Top with your choice of fresh berries, sliced fruits, nuts, coconut, chocolate chips, or any other toppings you prefer.

8. Serve chilled and enjoy your customizable Chia Seed Pudding!

Banana Ice Cream

Ingredients:
- 4 ripe bananas, peeled and sliced into coins
- 2 tablespoons honey or maple syrup (optional, for added sweetness)
- 1 teaspoon vanilla extract (optional, for flavor)
- Toppings (chocolate chips, nuts, fruit, etc., optional)

Instructions:
1. Slice the ripe bananas into coins and place them on a parchment-lined tray or plate. Make sure they are not touching each other.

2. Freeze the banana slices for at least 2-3 hours or until they are frozen solid. You can even freeze them overnight for best results.

3. Once the banana slices are frozen, transfer them to a food processor or high-speed blender.

4. Add honey or maple syrup and vanilla extract (if using) to the frozen banana slices.

5. Blend the mixture until smooth. You may need to stop and scrape down the sides of the processor or blender a few times to ensure even blending.

6. The banana mixture will go through stages of being crumbly and chunky before turning into a creamy ice cream consistency. Be patient, and keep blending until it's smooth and resembles soft-serve ice cream.

7. Taste the banana ice cream and adjust the sweetness or flavor as needed by adding more honey or vanilla extract.

8. If you'd like, fold in toppings such as chocolate chips, nuts, or fruit.

9. Serve the Banana Ice Cream immediately for a soft-serve texture or transfer it to an airtight container and freeze for a firmer ice cream.

Dark Chocolate-Dipped Strawberries

Ingredients:
- 1 pound fresh strawberries, washed and dried
- 8 ounces dark chocolate, chopped

- 1 tablespoon coconut oil (optional, for smoother chocolate)
- Toppings of your choice (e.g., chopped nuts, sprinkles, sea salt)

Instructions:

1. Prepare a baking sheet lined with parchment paper.

2. In a microwave-safe bowl, melt the dark chocolate in 30-second intervals, stirring each time until smooth. You can also melt the chocolate using a double boiler on the stove. If the chocolate seems too thick, you can add a tablespoon of coconut oil to thin it out for smoother dipping.

3. Hold a strawberry by the stem and dip it into the melted chocolate, swirling to coat it evenly. Allow any excess chocolate to drip back into the bowl.

4. Place the chocolate-dipped strawberry on the prepared baking sheet. If you're adding toppings like chopped nuts or sprinkles, do so immediately while the chocolate is still wet.

5. Repeat the dipping process with the remaining strawberries.

6. Let the chocolate-dipped strawberries cool and harden at room temperature or in the refrigerator for about 30 minutes.

7. Once the chocolate has set, your dark chocolate-dipped strawberries are ready to enjoy!

Oatmeal Cookies

Ingredients:
- 1 cup (2 sticks) unsalted butter, softened
- 1 cup granulated sugar
- 1 cup brown sugar, packed
- 2 large eggs
- 1 teaspoon pure vanilla extract
- 2 cups all-purpose flour
- 1 teaspoon baking soda
- 1 teaspoon ground cinnamon
- 1/2 teaspoon salt
- 3 cups old-fashioned rolled oats
- Optional: 1 cup of add-ins like chocolate chips, raisins, or chopped nuts

Instructions:
1. Preheat your oven to 350°F (175°C) and line a baking sheet with parchment paper.

2. In a large mixing bowl, cream together the softened butter, granulated sugar, and brown sugar until the mixture is light and fluffy.

3. Beat in the eggs one at a time, then stir in the vanilla extract.

4. In a separate bowl, whisk together the flour, baking soda, cinnamon, and salt.

5. Gradually add the dry ingredient mixture to the wet ingredients and mix until well combined.

6. Stir in the rolled oats and any optional add-ins (chocolate chips, raisins, nuts) of your choice.

7. Drop rounded tablespoons of cookie dough onto the prepared baking sheet, spacing them about 2 inches apart.

8. Bake in the preheated oven for 10 to 12 minutes, or until the edges are lightly golden but the centers are still soft.

9. Allow the cookies to cool on the baking sheet for a few minutes, then transfer them to a wire rack to cool completely.

10. Once cooled, your delicious oatmeal cookies are ready to enjoy!

Greek Yogurt with Honey and Nuts

Ingredients:

- 1 cup Greek yogurt
- 2 tablespoons honey (adjust to taste)
- 2 tablespoons chopped nuts (such as almonds, walnuts, or pistachios)
- Fresh fruit (optional, for garnish)

Instructions:

1. Start with a clean bowl or serving dish.
2. Spoon the Greek yogurt into the bowl or dish, spreading it evenly.
3. Drizzle the honey over the yogurt. You can adjust the amount of honey to suit your taste preferences, adding more for sweeter yogurt or less for a milder sweetness.
4. Sprinkle the chopped nuts evenly over the yogurt and honey.
5. If desired, you can garnish your Greek yogurt with fresh fruit, such as berries or sliced bananas.
6. Your Greek Yogurt with Honey and Nuts is ready to enjoy! You can either mix everything together before eating or enjoy the layers separately for different flavors and textures.

Baked Peaches

Ingredients:

- 4 ripe peaches
- 2 tablespoons butter, melted
- 2 tablespoons brown sugar (adjust to taste)
- 1/2 teaspoon ground cinnamon (adjust to taste)
- 1/4 teaspoon vanilla extract
- Optional toppings: Vanilla ice cream, whipped cream, chopped nuts, or a drizzle of honey

Instructions:

1. Preheat your oven to 375°F (190°C).
2. Wash the peaches, cut them in half, and remove the pits. You can also slice a small piece off the bottom of each peach half to make them more stable when baking.
3. Place the peach halves, cut side up, on a baking dish or a baking sheet lined with parchment paper.
4. In a small bowl, mix together the melted butter, brown sugar, ground cinnamon, and vanilla extract.
5. Spoon the buttery mixture over each peach half, making sure to drizzle it evenly.

6. Bake the peaches in the preheated oven for about 20-25 minutes or until they are tender and the tops have caramelized.

7. Remove the baked peaches from the oven and let them cool slightly before serving.

8. Serve your baked peaches on their own or with optional toppings like vanilla ice cream, whipped cream, chopped nuts, or a drizzle of honey.

Rice Pudding

Ingredients:

- 1 cup long-grain white rice
- 4 cups whole milk
- 1/2 cup granulated sugar (adjust to taste)
- 1/2 teaspoon salt
- 1 teaspoon vanilla extract
- 1/2 teaspoon ground cinnamon (optional)
- 1/2 cup raisins (optional)
- Ground nutmeg for garnish (optional)

Instructions:

1. Rinse the rice under cold water until the water runs clear. This helps remove excess starch.

2. In a large saucepan, combine the rinsed rice, milk, sugar, and salt. If you're using cinnamon, add it at this stage.

3. Place the saucepan over medium-high heat and bring the mixture to a boil, stirring frequently.

4. Once it starts boiling, reduce the heat to low and let it simmer. Cover the saucepan, but leave a small gap for steam to escape.

5. Simmer for about 30-40 minutes, or until the rice is tender and the mixture has thickened. Stir occasionally to prevent sticking.

6. If you're using raisins, add them in during the last 10 minutes of cooking.

7. Remove the saucepan from heat, and stir in the vanilla extract.

8. Let the rice pudding cool for a bit. It will continue to thicken as it cools.

9. If desired, sprinkle ground nutmeg on top for garnish.

10. Serve the rice pudding warm or chilled, depending on your preference.

Mango Sorbet

Ingredients:

- 4 ripe mangoes, peeled, pitted, and diced (about 4 cups)
- 1/2 cup granulated sugar (adjust to taste)
- 1/4 cup freshly squeezed lime or lemon juice (about 2 limes or lemons)
- 1/4 cup water
- A pinch of salt

Instructions:

1. Place the diced mangoes in a blender or food processor.
2. Add the granulated sugar, lime or lemon juice, water, and a pinch of salt to the blender.
3. Blend the mixture until it becomes smooth and creamy. You may need to scrape down the sides of the blender or food processor and blend again to ensure a uniform consistency.
4. Taste the mixture and adjust the sweetness by adding more sugar if needed. Keep in mind that the sweetness will be slightly muted once the sorbet is frozen.
5. Once you're satisfied with the taste, transfer the mango mixture to an ice cream maker.

6. Churn the mixture in the ice cream maker according to the manufacturer's instructions. This typically takes about 20-30 minutes.

7. After churning, the sorbet should have a soft-serve consistency. You can enjoy it immediately if you prefer a softer texture, or transfer it to an airtight container and freeze for a few hours for a firmer texture.

8. Scoop and serve your homemade mango sorbet as a delightful, tropical dessert!

Frozen Yogurt Bark

Ingredients:
- 2 cups Greek yogurt (any flavor you like)
- 2-3 tablespoons honey or maple syrup (adjust to taste)
- 1/2 cup fresh berries (e.g., strawberries, blueberries, raspberries)
- 1/4 cup granola
- 1/4 cup chopped nuts (e.g., almonds, walnuts) (optional)
- A pinch of cinnamon (optional)

Instructions:

1. Line a baking sheet or shallow dish with parchment paper. Make sure it fits in your freezer.

2. In a bowl, mix the Greek yogurt and honey or maple syrup until well combined. Adjust the sweetness to your taste.

3. Spread the sweetened yogurt mixture evenly onto the parchment paper in a rectangular or square shape, about 1/4 to 1/2 inch thick.

4. Sprinkle the fresh berries, granola, and chopped nuts (if using) evenly over the yogurt.

5. Optionally, dust the top with a pinch of cinnamon for extra flavor.

6. Carefully place the baking sheet or dish in the freezer.

7. Freeze for at least 2-3 hours, or until the yogurt bark is completely frozen.

8. Once frozen, remove the yogurt bark from the freezer and break it into pieces using your hands or a knife.

9. Serve immediately, and enjoy your frozen yogurt bark as a delicious and nutritious snack!

Mixed Berries with Whipped Cream

Ingredients:

- 2 cups mixed berries (strawberries, blueberries, raspberries, blackberries, etc.)
- 1 cup heavy whipping cream
- 2 tablespoons powdered sugar (adjust to taste)
- 1 teaspoon vanilla extract
- Fresh mint leaves for garnish (optional)

Instructions:

1. Wash the mixed berries and gently pat them dry with a paper towel. You can use any combination of berries you like or have on hand.
2. In a mixing bowl, combine the heavy whipping cream, powdered sugar, and vanilla extract.
3. Use a hand mixer or stand mixer to whip the cream until it forms stiff peaks. This will take a few minutes. Be careful not to over-whip; stop as soon as stiff peaks form.
4. Spoon a generous portion of the whipped cream onto serving plates or into dessert bowls.
5. Arrange the mixed berries on top of the whipped cream.
6. Optionally, garnish with fresh mint leaves for added flavor and a pop of color.

7. Serve your mixed berries with whipped cream immediately and enjoy!

Peanut Butter and Banana Sandwich

Ingredients:
- 2 slices of bread (white, whole wheat, or your choice)
- 2-3 tablespoons peanut butter (smooth or crunchy, as you prefer)
- 1 ripe banana, peeled and sliced
- Honey or a drizzle of maple syrup (optional, for extra sweetness)
- A pinch of cinnamon (optional)

Instructions:
1. Lay out the two slices of bread on a clean surface.
2. Spread peanut butter evenly on one or both slices of bread, depending on your preference for peanut butter coverage.
3. Place the banana slices on one slice of bread. If you like, you can sprinkle a pinch of cinnamon over the banana slices for extra flavor.

4. If you want to add sweetness, drizzle honey or maple syrup over the banana slices. This step is optional, as the natural sweetness of ripe bananas pairs well with peanut butter.

5. Place the other slice of bread on top to form a sandwich.

6. Press the two halves together gently.

7. Optionally, you can cut the sandwich in half diagonally for easier handling.

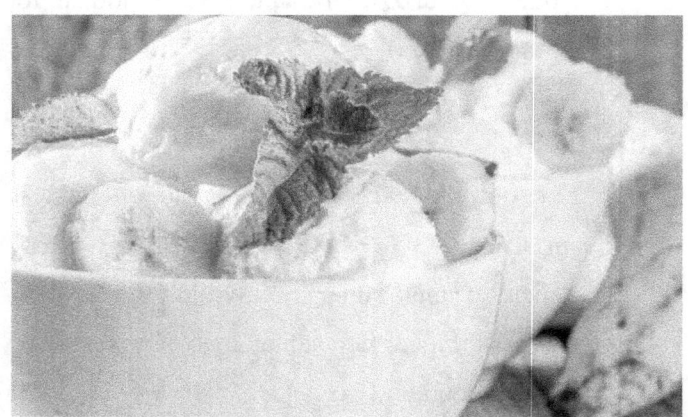

CHAPTER 13: SMOOTHIES

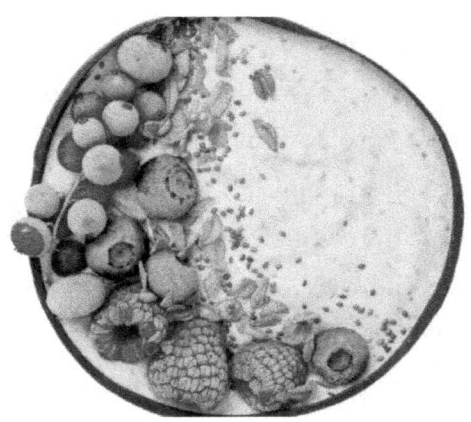

Berry Blast Smoothie

Ingredients:

- 1 cup mixed berries (strawberries, blueberries, raspberries, blackberries)
- 1 ripe banana
- 1/2 cup Greek yogurt (plain or flavored)
- 1/2 cup milk (dairy or plant-based)
- 1 tablespoon honey or maple syrup (optional, for added sweetness)
- 1/2 cup ice cubes (optional, for a colder and thicker smoothie)

Instructions:

1. Place the mixed berries, ripe banana, Greek yogurt, and milk in a blender.
2. If you'd like a sweeter smoothie, you can add honey or maple syrup at this point. Adjust the sweetness to your taste.
3. Optionally, add ice cubes to make the smoothie colder and thicker. This is especially nice on hot days.
4. Blend all the ingredients until smooth and creamy. You may need to stop and scrape down the sides of the blender and blend again to ensure everything is well mixed.
5. Once the smoothie has reached your desired consistency, pour it into a glass.
6. If you'd like, garnish with a few fresh berries or a mint leaf for an extra touch of freshness.
7. Serve your Berry Blast Smoothie immediately and enjoy!

Green Detox Smoothie

Ingredients:

- 1 cup fresh spinach leaves
- 1/2 cucumber, peeled and chopped

- 1/2 green apple, cored and chopped
- 1 celery stalk, chopped
- 1/2 lemon, juiced
- 1/2 cup water or coconut water (adjust for desired consistency)
- 1 teaspoon honey or maple syrup (optional, for sweetness)
- Ice cubes (optional, for a colder smoothie)

Instructions:

1. Place the fresh spinach, chopped cucumber, green apple, celery, and lemon juice in a blender.
2. Add water or coconut water to the blender to help with blending. Adjust the amount based on how thick or thin you want your smoothie.
3. If you'd like your smoothie to be sweeter, you can add a teaspoon of honey or maple syrup at this point. Taste and adjust as needed.
4. If you prefer a colder smoothie, you can add a few ice cubes to the blender.
5. Blend all the ingredients until you achieve a smooth and creamy consistency. You may need to stop and scrape down the sides of the blender to ensure everything is well mixed.

6. Once your Green Detox Smoothie is ready, pour it into a glass.

7. Optionally, you can garnish with a slice of lemon or a sprig of mint for a refreshing touch.

8. Serve your smoothie immediately and enjoy the detoxifying goodness!

Tropical Paradise Smoothie

Ingredients:
- 1 cup frozen mango chunks
- 1/2 cup frozen pineapple chunks
- 1 ripe banana
- 1/2 cup coconut milk (or coconut water for a lighter option)
- 1/2 cup plain Greek yogurt
- 1 tablespoon honey or maple syrup (adjust to taste)
- 1/2 cup orange juice
- Ice cubes (optional, for extra chill)

Instructions:
1. Place the frozen mango chunks, frozen pineapple chunks, ripe banana, coconut milk, plain Greek yogurt, honey or maple syrup, and orange juice in a blender.

2. If you prefer your smoothie to be colder, you can add a few ice cubes to the blender.

3. Blend all the ingredients until you achieve a smooth and creamy consistency. You may need to stop and scrape down the sides of the blender to ensure everything is well mixed.

4. Taste the smoothie and adjust the sweetness with more honey or maple syrup if desired.

5. Once your Tropical Paradise Smoothie is ready, pour it into a glass.

6. Optionally, you can garnish it with a slice of fresh pineapple or a maraschino cherry for a tropical flair.

7. Serve your smoothie immediately and enjoy your taste of paradise!

Banana Almond Butter Smoothie

Ingredients:
- 1 ripe banana
- 2 tablespoons almond butter
- 1 cup almond milk (or your preferred milk)
- 1/2 cup plain Greek yogurt (or dairy-free alternative)

- 1 tablespoon honey or maple syrup (adjust to taste)
- 1/2 teaspoon ground cinnamon (optional)
- Ice cubes (optional, for extra chill)

Instructions:

1. Peel the ripe banana and place it in a blender.
2. Add the almond butter, almond milk, plain Greek yogurt, honey or maple syrup, and ground cinnamon (if using) to the blender.
3. If you prefer a colder smoothie, you can add a few ice cubes to the blender as well.
4. Blend all the ingredients until the mixture is smooth and creamy. You may need to stop and scrape down the sides of the blender to ensure everything is well mixed.
5. Taste the smoothie and adjust the sweetness with more honey or maple syrup if needed.
6. Once your Banana Almond Butter Smoothie is ready, pour it into a glass.
7. Optionally, you can garnish with a sprinkle of ground cinnamon or a drizzle of almond butter for added flavor.
8. Serve your smoothie immediately and enjoy the creamy, nutty goodness!

Beet and Berry Smoothie

Ingredients:

- 1 small beet, peeled and diced (you can use cooked or raw, but cooked beets are easier to blend)
- 1 cup mixed berries (strawberries, blueberries, raspberries)
- 1 ripe banana
- 1 cup spinach leaves (optional, for added greens)
- 1/2 cup Greek yogurt (plain or flavored)
- 1/2 cup water or coconut water (adjust for desired consistency)
- 1 tablespoon honey or maple syrup (adjust to taste)
- Ice cubes (optional, for a colder smoothie)

Instructions:

1. If you're using a raw beet, make sure to peel and dice it into smaller pieces to help with blending. If you have cooked beets on hand, you can skip this step.

2. Place the diced beet (cooked or raw), mixed berries, ripe banana, spinach leaves (if using), Greek yogurt, honey or maple syrup, and water or coconut water in a blender.

3. If you prefer your smoothie to be colder, you can add a few ice cubes to the blender.

4. Blend all the ingredients until you achieve a smooth and vibrant pinkish-purple color. You may need to stop and scrape down the sides of the blender to ensure everything is well mixed.

5. Taste the smoothie and adjust the sweetness with more honey or maple syrup if desired.

6. Once your Beet and Berry Smoothie is ready, pour it into a glass.

7. Serve your smoothie immediately and enjoy the sweet and earthy flavors!

Spinach and Pineapple Smoothie

Ingredients:
- 1 cup fresh spinach leaves
- 1 cup frozen pineapple chunks
- 1 ripe banana
- 1/2 cup Greek yogurt (plain or flavored)
- 1/2 cup water or coconut water (adjust for desired consistency)
- 1 tablespoon honey or maple syrup (adjust to taste)
- Ice cubes (optional, for a colder smoothie)

Instructions:

1. Place the fresh spinach leaves, frozen pineapple chunks, ripe banana, Greek yogurt, honey or maple syrup, and water or coconut water in a blender.

2. If you prefer your smoothie to be colder, you can add a few ice cubes to the blender.

3. Blend all the ingredients until you achieve a smooth and vibrant green color. You may need to stop and scrape down the sides of the blender to ensure everything is well mixed.

4. Taste the smoothie and adjust the sweetness with more honey or maple syrup if desired.

5. Once your Spinach and Pineapple Smoothie is ready, pour it into a glass.

6. Serve your smoothie immediately and enjoy the tropical, green goodness!

Chia Seed and Coconut Smoothie

Ingredients:

- 2 tablespoons chia seeds
- 1 cup coconut milk (canned or carton, unsweetened)
- 1 ripe banana

- 1/2 cup Greek yogurt (plain or flavored)
- 1 tablespoon honey or maple syrup (adjust to taste)
- 1/2 teaspoon vanilla extract
- Ice cubes (optional, for a colder smoothie)
- Shredded coconut for garnish (optional)

Instructions:

1. In a small bowl, combine the chia seeds and coconut milk. Stir well to ensure the chia seeds are evenly distributed in the milk. Allow this mixture to sit for about 10-15 minutes, or until it thickens and forms a gel-like consistency. This is your chia seed pudding base.

2. In a blender, place the ripe banana, Greek yogurt, honey or maple syrup, vanilla extract, and ice cubes (if using).

3. Add the chia seed pudding mixture to the blender.

4. Blend all the ingredients until you achieve a smooth and creamy consistency. You may need to stop and scrape down the sides of the blender to ensure everything is well mixed.

5. Taste the smoothie and adjust the sweetness with more honey or maple syrup if desired.

6. Once your Chia Seed and Coconut Smoothie is ready, pour it into a glass.

7. Optionally, garnish with shredded coconut for extra coconut flavor and texture.

8. Serve your smoothie immediately and enjoy the creamy and nutritious goodness!

Avocado and Spinach Smoothie

Ingredients:

- 1 ripe avocado, peeled and pitted
- 1 cup fresh spinach leaves
- 1 banana
- 1 cup milk (dairy or plant-based)
- 1/2 cup Greek yogurt (plain or flavored)
- 1 tablespoon honey or maple syrup (adjust to taste)
- Ice cubes (optional, for a colder smoothie)

Instructions:

1. In a blender, place the ripe avocado, fresh spinach leaves, banana, milk, Greek yogurt, honey or maple syrup, and ice cubes (if using).

2. Blend all the ingredients until you achieve a smooth and creamy consistency.

3. You may need to stop and scrape down the sides of the blender to ensure everything is well mixed.

4. Taste the smoothie and adjust the sweetness with more honey or maple syrup if desired.

5. Once your Avocado and Spinach Smoothie is ready, pour it into a glass.

6. Serve your smoothie immediately and enjoy the creamy and green goodness!

Mango Turmeric Smoothie

Ingredients:
- 1 cup frozen mango chunks
- 1 ripe banana
- 1/2 cup Greek yogurt (plain or flavored)
- 1/2 cup milk (dairy or plant-based)
- 1/2 teaspoon ground turmeric
- 1/2 teaspoon ground ginger
- 1 tablespoon honey or maple syrup (adjust to taste)
- A pinch of black pepper (optional, enhances turmeric absorption)
- Ice cubes (optional, for a colder smoothie)

Instructions:

1. Place the frozen mango chunks, ripe banana, Greek yogurt, milk, ground turmeric, ground ginger, honey or maple syrup, and a pinch of black pepper (if using) in a blender.
2. If you prefer your smoothie to be colder, you can add a few ice cubes to the blender as well.
3. Blend all the ingredients until you achieve a smooth and vibrant yellow color. You may need to stop and scrape down the sides of the blender to ensure everything is well mixed.
4. Taste the smoothie and adjust the sweetness with more honey or maple syrup if desired.
5. Once your Mango Turmeric Smoothie is ready, pour it into a glass.
6. Serve your smoothie immediately and enjoy the tropical, turmeric goodness!

Peach and Oat Smoothie

Ingredients:

- 1 cup fresh or frozen peach slices
- 1/2 cup rolled oats
- 1 ripe banana
- 1/2 cup Greek yogurt (plain or flavored)

- 1/2 cup milk (dairy or plant-based)
- 1 tablespoon honey or maple syrup (adjust to taste)
- Ice cubes (optional, for a colder smoothie)

Instructions:

1. Place the peach slices, rolled oats, ripe banana, Greek yogurt, milk, honey or maple syrup, and ice cubes (if using) in a blender.
2. Blend all the ingredients until you achieve a smooth and creamy consistency. You may need to stop and scrape down the sides of the blender to ensure everything is well mixed.
3. Taste the smoothie and adjust the sweetness with more honey or maple syrup if desired.
4. Once your Peach and Oat Smoothie is ready, pour it into a glass.
5. Serve your smoothie immediately and enjoy the peachy and hearty goodness!

Blueberry Flaxseed Smoothie

Ingredients:

- 1 cup frozen blueberries
- 1 ripe banana

- 1 cup unsweetened almond milk (or any milk of your choice)
- 1 tablespoon ground flaxseeds
- 1 tablespoon honey (optional for sweetness)
- 1/2 cup Greek yogurt (optional for creaminess)
- Ice cubes (optional for a colder smoothie)

Instructions:

1. Add the frozen blueberries, ripe banana, almond milk, ground flaxseeds, honey (if desired), and Greek yogurt (if using) to a blender.
2. Blend all the ingredients until smooth. If you prefer a thicker consistency, you can add more frozen blueberries or ice cubes.
3. Taste the smoothie and adjust the sweetness or thickness to your liking by adding more honey or almond milk if needed.
4. Once you're satisfied with the texture and taste, pour the smoothie into a glass and enjoy!

Chocolate Banana Smoothie

Ingredients:

- 2 ripe bananas
- 1 cup milk (or a dairy-free alternative like almond or soy milk)

- 2 tablespoons cocoa powder
- 2 tablespoons honey or maple syrup (adjust to taste)
- 1/2 cup Greek yogurt (optional for creaminess)
- 1/2 teaspoon vanilla extract
- Ice cubes (optional for a colder smoothie)

Instructions:

1. Peel and slice the ripe bananas.
2. In a blender, combine the sliced bananas, milk, cocoa powder, honey or maple syrup, Greek yogurt (if using), and vanilla extract.
3. Add ice cubes if you prefer a colder smoothie or want to make it thicker.
4. Blend all the ingredients until smooth and creamy. You can adjust the sweetness by adding more honey or cocoa powder to taste.
5. Once your Chocolate Banana Smoothie reaches your desired consistency and flavor, pour it into a glass.
6. Optionally, you can garnish your smoothie with a drizzle of chocolate syrup, chocolate shavings, or a banana slice.
7. Enjoy your creamy and chocolaty delight!

Carrot and Ginger Smoothie

Ingredients:

- 2 medium-sized carrots, peeled and chopped
- 1-inch piece of fresh ginger, peeled and minced (adjust to taste)
- 1 cup orange juice (freshly squeezed is best)
- 1/2 cup Greek yogurt (optional for creaminess)
- 1 tablespoon honey or maple syrup (adjust to taste)
- Ice cubes (optional for a colder smoothie)

Instructions:

1. Prepare the carrots by peeling and chopping them into smaller pieces for easier blending.
2. Peel and mince the fresh ginger. You can adjust the amount of ginger based on your preference for spiciness.
3. In a blender, combine the chopped carrots, minced ginger, orange juice, Greek yogurt (if using), and honey or maple syrup.
4. Add ice cubes if you want a colder and thicker smoothie.
5. Blend all the ingredients until smooth and well combined.

6. Taste the smoothie and adjust the sweetness or spiciness by adding more honey, ginger, or orange juice if desired.
7. Once your Carrot and Ginger Smoothie reaches your desired flavor and consistency, pour it into a glass.
8. Optionally, you can garnish your smoothie with a sprinkle of ground cinnamon or a slice of fresh orange.
9. Enjoy your healthy and invigorating Carrot and Ginger Smoothie!

Papaya and Lime Smoothie

Ingredients:
- 1 cup ripe papaya, peeled, seeded, and cubed
- Juice of 1 lime
- 1/2 cup plain yogurt (or dairy-free yogurt for a vegan option)
- 1-2 tablespoons honey or maple syrup (adjust to taste)
- Ice cubes (optional for a colder smoothie)
- Fresh mint leaves for garnish (optional)

Instructions:

1. Peel, seed, and cube the ripe papaya. Make sure it's ripe for the best flavor.

2. Squeeze the juice from one lime.

3. In a blender, combine the cubed papaya, lime juice, plain yogurt, and honey or maple syrup.

4. Add ice cubes if you want a colder and thicker smoothie.

5. Blend all the ingredients until smooth and creamy. Taste the smoothie and adjust the sweetness or tartness by adding more honey or lime juice if desired.

6. Once your Papaya and Lime Smoothie reaches your desired flavor and consistency, pour it into a glass.

7. Optionally, garnish your smoothie with fresh mint leaves for a burst of freshness.

8. Enjoy your tropical and zesty Papaya and Lime Smoothie!

"Every positive choice I make contributes to my liver's well-being."

"I am surrounded by the support and energy needed for my liver to thrive."

CONCLUSION

In conclusion, the "Fatty Liver Diet Cookbook for Newly Diagnosed" is a thorough and helpful resource for people dealing with fatty liver disease. This precisely designed guide not only educates readers on the need of a liver-friendly diet, but also provides them with a wide range of nutritious dishes.

The cookbook stands out for its approachable nature, with clear and simple instructions for making meals that improve liver function. The addition of a 30-day meal plan increases its usefulness by providing a structured route to reaching optimal well-being. This strategic strategy not only provides a varied and balanced diet, but it also makes incorporating liver-revitalizing meals into one's daily routine easier.

Aside from its culinary offers, the book delves into the complexities of controlling fatty liver disease, promoting a comprehensive awareness of the lifestyle modifications required for long-term liver health. The emphasis on nutrient-dense products and mindful dining throughout the cookbook, reinforcing the cookbook's commitment to liver revitalization and general health.

In essence, the "Fatty Liver Diet Cookbook for Newly Diagnosed" is more than just a cookbook; it is a handbook that enables people to take control of their health journey. This cookbook emerges as a necessary companion for anyone looking to embrace a liver-friendly lifestyle and embark on a path to holistic well-being by combining expert insights, practical meal planning, and tasty recipes.

HAPPY COOKING!

WEEKLY MEAL PLANNER

MONDAY	TUESDAY	WEDNESDAY

THURSDAY	FRIDAY	SHOPPING LIST

SATURDAY	SUNDAY	

Notes:

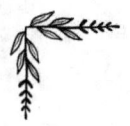

WEEKLY MEAL PLANNER

MONDAY	TUESDAY	WEDNESDAY

THURSDAY	FRIDAY	SHOPPING LIST

SATURDAY	SUNDAY

Notes:

WEEKLY MEAL PLANNER

MONDAY	TUESDAY	WEDNESDAY

THURSDAY	FRIDAY

SHOPPING LIST

_____
_____
_____
_____
_____
_____

SATURDAY	SUNDAY

_____
_____
_____
_____
_____
_____
_____

Notes:

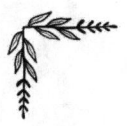

WEEKLY MEAL PLANNER

MONDAY	TUESDAY	WEDNESDAY

THURSDAY	FRIDAY	**SHOPPING LIST**

SATURDAY	SUNDAY

Notes:

WEEKLY MEAL PLANNER

MONDAY	TUESDAY	WEDNESDAY

THURSDAY	FRIDAY	SHOPPING LIST

SATURDAY	SUNDAY

Notes:

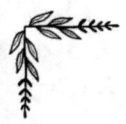

WEEKLY MEAL PLANNER

MONDAY	TUESDAY	WEDNESDAY

THURSDAY	FRIDAY	SHOPPING LIST

SATURDAY	SUNDAY

Notes:

329

WEEKLY MEAL PLANNER

MONDAY	TUESDAY	WEDNESDAY

THURSDAY	FRIDAY	SHOPPING LIST

SATURDAY	SUNDAY

Notes:

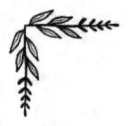

WEEKLY MEAL PLANNER

MONDAY	TUESDAY	WEDNESDAY

THURSDAY	FRIDAY

SHOPPING LIST

SATURDAY	SUNDAY

Notes:

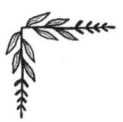

WEEKLY MEAL PLANNER

MONDAY	TUESDAY	WEDNESDAY

THURSDAY	FRIDAY	SHOPPING LIST

SATURDAY	SUNDAY

Notes:

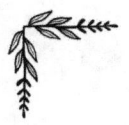

WEEKLY MEAL PLANNER

MONDAY	TUESDAY	WEDNESDAY

THURSDAY	FRIDAY	SHOPPING LIST

SATURDAY	SUNDAY

Notes:

www.ingramcontent.com/pod-product-compliance
Lightning Source LLC
Chambersburg PA
CBHW071201290526
45796CB00008B/93